Practical Aspects of
MENTAL HEALTH
CONSULTATION

Practical Aspects of
MENTAL HEALTH
CONSULTATION

Edited by

JACK ZUSMAN, M.D.

Professor of Psychiatry and Director
Division of Community Psychiatry
School of Medicine
State University of New York at Buffalo

DAVID L. DAVIDSON, M.D.

Formerly Assistant Professor of Psychiatry
School of Medicine
State University of New York at Buffalo

With an Introduction by

Peter F. Regan, M.D.

Professor of Psychiatry
School of Medicine
State University of New York at Buffalo

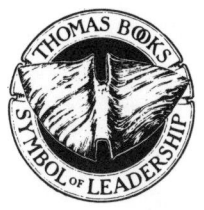

CHARLES C THOMAS • PUBLISHER
Springfield • Illinois • U.S.A.

Published and Distributed Throughout the World by
CHARLES C THOMAS • PUBLISHER
Bannerstone House
301-327 East Lawrence Avenue, Springfield, Illinois, U.S.A.
Natchez Plantation House
735 North Atlantic Boulevard, Fort Lauderdale, Florida, U.S.A.

©*1972, by* CHARLES C THOMAS • PUBLISHER
ISBN 0-398-02449-9
Library of Congress Catalog Card Number: 77-184618

Printed in the United States of America
RN-1

CONTRIBUTORS

HAROUTUN M. BABIGIAN, M.D.

Associate Professor of Psychiatry and Director
Division of Preventive and Social Psychiatry
Department of Psychiatry
The University of Rochester
School of Medicine and Dentistry
Rochester, New York

JOHN H. BEARD, M.S.W.

Executive Director
Fountain House
New York, New York

DAVID L. DAVIDSON, M.D.

Formerly Assistant Professor of Psychiatry
School of Medicine
State University of New York at Buffalo
Buffalo, New York

JUDITH A. FALCONER, M.A.

Assistant to Chairman
Department of Biochemistry
State University of New York at Buffalo
Buffalo, New York

GERTRUDE E. FLYNN, R.N., M.S.

Professor and Associate Director
Psychiatric Nursing Service
University of Rochester Medical Center
Rochester, New York

ANTHONY M. GRAZIANO, Ph.D.

Associate Professor of Psychology
Faculty of Social Sciences and Administration
State University of New York at Buffalo
Buffalo, New York

MURRAY LEVINE, Ph.D.

Professor and Director
Professional Psychology Area
Department of Psychology
Faculty of Social Sciences and Administration
State University of New York at Buffalo
Buffalo, New York

ANDREAS M. PEDERSON, Ph.D.

Assistant Professor of Psychiatry and Psychology
Department of Psychiatry
University of Rochester
School of Medicine and Dentistry
Rochester, New York

QUENTIN RAE-GRANT, M.D.

Professor of Child Psychiatry
Psychiatrist-in-Chief
The Hospital for Sick Children
Toronto, Ontario, Canada

PETER F. REGAN, M.D.

Professor of Psychiatry
School of Medicine
State University of New York at Buffalo
Buffalo, New York

JAMES A. ROBINSON, M.D.

Assistant Professor of Psychiatry
School of Medicine
State University of New York at Buffalo
Buffalo, New York

ZEBULON C. TAINTOR, M.D.

Assistant Professor of Psychiatry
School of Medicine
State University of New York at Buffalo
Buffalo, New York

JACK ZUSMAN, M.D.

*Professor of Psychiatry and Director
Division of Community Psychiatry
School of Medicine
State University of New York at Buffalo
Buffalo, New York*

PREFACE

THIS book results from the second annual Division of Community Psychiatry conference held in January, 1970, at the State University of New York at Buffalo. These conferences, which are part of a larger Continuing Medical Education project sponsored by the Departments of Psychiatry and Continuing Medical Education, are presented once a year to bring together experts on a particular aspect of community mental health practice. The material in the present volume is based upon most of the papers presented at the conference on "Mental Health Consultation."

I want to express my thanks to the staff of Continuing Medical Education (Harry J. Alvis, M.D., formerly Director and Associate Dean for Continuing Medical Education) and of the Department of Psychiatry (S. Mouchly Small, M.D., Professor and Chairman) for their help in organizing and carrying out the conference. The conference itself was supported financially in part by Grant No. 11334 from the National Institute of Mental Health of the Department of Health, Education, and Welfare, and by the New York State Department of Mental Hygiene. The preparation of the present volume has been greatly assisted by Miss Phyllis Zusman.

JACK ZUSMAN

INTRODUCTION

G. K. CHESTERTON, that master of paradox, would have revelled in the opportunity to examine community psychiatry. For here is a field beset with paradoxes, and yet a field so vital that incongruities must be tolerated and maintained.

In many ways, the very name "community psychiatry" summarizes the paradoxes.

On the one hand, community psychiatry must be psychiatric. As such, it must come to grips with the infinitely variable needs of the millions of individuals suffering from mental illness, and the many millions of individuals burdened by partial mental or emotional impairment. Any student of psychiatry will recognize that each of these individuals is unique, and that the process of improving his or her adaptability and pleasure in life is equally unique. The wisdom accumulated in centuries of psychological medicine makes it clear that such an individualized treatment process is dependent upon human contact of a personal, respectful, humane, and understanding sort.

So "psychiatry" must reject pat formulations, and must demand personal interaction with each afflicted and near-afflicted person.

But the "community" part of community psychiatry is driven to general programs and remoteness. Even if one takes with a grain of salt the assertion that one person in ten is afflicted with mental illness, the numbers of mentally ill people far outstrip the capacities of highly trained specialists to provide individual care. The many millions more who suffer partial disabilities are clearly unable to obtain individual help from the mental health specialists. Moreover, evidence points to the fact that the afflicted and near-afflicted can suffer or gain from the actions and attitudes of the many who are "well," and these are clearly far beyond approach by the highly trained specialist.

The community, therefore, must find a set of general measures and approaches which will bring about the individual therapeutic contact that psychiatry demands, while simultaneously altering the milieu in a salutary fashion hopefully leading to decreases in the numbers who reach the stage where individualized and highly personal contacts are of the essence.

To create a communitywide program which yet retains its individuality; to recognize the manpower limits of highly specialized mental health personnel, and yet to bring their sophistication to countless millions of sufferers; to provide an orderly approach, and yet cultivate pluralism: these are the paradoxical aims that must be somehow contained by the field of community psychiatry. It is this very richness of paradox which would have fascinated Chesterton . . . and the quasi-religious fervor which can sometimes be found among community psychiatrists would have added to his zest!

In order to contain the paradox, community psychiatry must grapple with three monumental needs.

In the first instance, community psychiatry needs general theories, and it is not yet ready for them. It is still laboring through a reductionistic period of investigation. While there have been a few attempts to mount general theories, these have fallen by the wayside because of ineffectiveness, limited applicability, and insufficient information. The field of community psychiatry is still in that state in which the accumulation of new information, and the gradual ordering of that new information into more and more comprehensive formulations, must be pursued with patience and dedication.

Secondly, community psychiatry must learn to deal with social perceptions, both within the field of medicine and in society at large. Just as preventive medicine has found that it must persuade people to make use of techniques like immunization or knowledge like the harmful consequences of smoking, and just as nutritional experts must persuade a population to use new methods of agriculture and fertilization, so also is community psychiatry confronted with the need to persuade on those issues where knowledge has been accumulated. It does little good simply to know that certain sets of social situations predispose to breakdown, unless means are found for persuading individuals, communities, and governments to alter those dangerous conditions.

Finally, community psychiatry must in some fashion find a way of delimiting its sphere of expertise, so that it can work in close collaboration with other disciplines as disciplines. At the moment, a dozen primrose paths seem to lead the community psychiatrists further and further away from their own basic area of expertise, until they find themselves in the swamplands of economics, or construction, or politics. Away from their own field, they are too frequently novices, and their amateurish efforts can imperil the validity of psychiatrically sound expertise.

So there are needs which reverberate within the general paradox: a need for the accumulation of information, a need to persuade society to act on the basis of information, a need for the field itself to discover a firmer base of operations. And with all of these needs satisfied, the essential paradox of being simultaneously generalized and individualized will still remain to be mastered.

In considering any new development in community psychiatry, therefore, one attempts to assess the degree to which it will satisfy these needs and help to master this paradox. Will the development add to knowledge? Will it help to find new means of persuading society? Will it help to define better the field of community psychiatry? Will it bridge the gap between the general and the particular?

To all of these questions, a reader of this volume will discover affirmative answers. By focusing attention on the process of consultation, the authors have made a number of contributions, perhaps in more ways than they had originally intended. The essence of this contribution, it seems to me, is the repeated thrust toward a bipolar mode of consultation. As one pursues the material in chapter after chapter, one comes to recognize more and more clearly that what is being described is a two-way process: wisdom is going in both directions, and both the consultant and the consultee are the beneficiaries.

This bipolar mode of consultation has clear implications for mastering the paradox between the generalized and the individualized; it provides a constant feedback mechanism for adjusting general directions to the unique needs of individuals, even as it multiplies the capacities of the mental health specialist to deal with the community's population. The same reverberating effect can serve as an "early warning system," alerting the specialist when he is beginning to exceed the limits of his expertise, and thus helping further to define the nature of the field of community psychiatry. In the very process of persuading consultees, and guiding them in persuading others, more and more knowledge about how to change society's perceptions and actions will undoubtedly accrue.

In evaluating the many possible positive implications of this volume, however, one must not mistake enthusiasm for grandiosity. At root, this work contributes to the first need of the field of community psychiatry: the need for more information. It is a contribution, in every sense of the word; it is an addition to our knowledge, but by no means a completion.

It is just this painstaking analysis of crucial phenomena, carefully executed, that will bring about a sufficient body of knowledge so that our actions will become more expert and more effective. More than fifteen years ago, Alexander Leighton, in an informal discussion, pointed out that workers in the field of social psychiatry had to be content with "gnawing away at the mountain, rather like mice." The analogy is not flattering, but it is curiously felicitous. In the intervening years, the patient accumulation of information by Leighton and others has made the mountain smaller, and the present volume will help the process.

The present volume, then, is a specific and valuable contribution to our knowledge of the field of community psychiatry, as well as being a useful set of guidelines for those who are daily confronted with the need to match their expertise against the overwhelming demands of the communities in which they work.

PETER F. REGAN

CONTENTS

Practical Aspects of
**MENTAL HEALTH
CONSULTATION**

SECTION I
Theory of
Mental Health Consultation

INTRODUCTION

THIS book, devoted to practical aspects of mental health consultation, nevertheless begins with two chapters on mental health consultation theory. The reader may well ask why.

Professional practice and especially mental health professional practice has often been overburdened with theory to the point where concern with theory crowded out service. Yet, the opposite situation — an absence of theory with complete concentration on service — is just as unfortunate. Some theoretical structure — that is, an abstract description of what happens and why — is absolutely necessary. Without it, each situation is unique, there is no carry-over from one experience to the next, and teaching becomes impossible. A theory of consultation facilitates description of the interaction between the mental health consultant and his consultee. The theory permits generalizations to be made and helps the consultant to organize his experience and recognize similarities from one consultation situation to the next. The theory assists the consultant in determining what to do when he otherwise would be uncertain. Even if the theory is wrong, it helps to allay the anxiety of the consultant and in this way at least, quite likely has a facilitating effect on the consultee. The theory predicts the outcome of any particular consultation situation and makes it possible when an unexpected outcome occurs to consider what particular factor or factors led to the unanticipated developments.

Without a theory, it is hardly possible to test the effectiveness of consultation or to improve technique. In any situation of interaction between two individuals there is an infinite number of variables which could be studied. It is the theory which suggests the important variables and directs the researcher to focus on changes in these variables.

Mental health consultation has developed in large part from a psychoanalytic foundation. Gerald Caplan, a psychoanalyst, has been one of the most influential practitioners. Moreover, in the past twenty years during which mental health consultation was becoming an important aspect of mental health practice, most mental health practitioners have had strong backgrounds in analytic theory and practice. It was natural, then, that early mental health consultation theory emphasize psychodynamics and unconscious factors in the consultee. Theme interference, as discussed by Caplan (1970), is certainly closely related to, if not the same as countertransference.

In the following two chapters, some theoretical bases of mental health consultation are proposed from a new point of view. Both Levine and Zusman are members of what might be called the second postwar generation of mental health professionals − those who were influenced by psychoanalytic approaches but who have tended to deemphasize psychoanalysis and instead concentrate on social interactional and situational factors. Both Levine and Zusman approach consultation from a concern with problems of bureaucracy and of social welfare organizations and an awareness of the power of these organizations to influence those whom they serve. Both authors see the consultants, the consultees, and the clients as actors in a social drama, each playing out very well-defined roles.

It is very striking that although the backgrounds of these two authors are rather dissimilar (one with a Ph.D. in psychology and extensive experience working with school systems and other services for children, the other with an M.D. and training in psychiatry and public health), they come up with similar questions and similar proposals for answers. They are both concerned with social labeling and its effects on clients. They both emphasize the opportunity the consultant has to influence the labeling process and the difference the consultant's intervention in this process can mean for the client. They both point out the general social role of the consultant regardless of his particular skills as a mental health professional. They deemphasize the differences among the mental health professions and seem to see the consultant as a jack-of-all-trades who often steps in to do what needs to be done. They both accept bureaucracy as a fact of life and seem to feel that the consultant must be a master at manipulation of the bureaucracy.

Levine in particular emphasizes what might be called "the antiparanoid view"; that is, he sees problems which require the intervention of the consultant resulting not from any individual's deliberate or unconscious negative actions but rather from an unfortunate combination of circumstances. He sees the consultees — the caretakers — struggling against overwhelming difficulties produced by problems of organization and shortages of resources. The consultant's role, then, is to deal with these organizational problems and relieve some of the pressures on the consultee but not necessarily to produce any change in the consultee.

Another aspect of Levine's work worth noting is his historical point of view. This is a rare commodity among modern mental health professionals. The mental health professional who examines the historical foundations of his work is likely to be shocked and perhaps chagrined to find that the issues he considers timely and the battles he is presently fighting were modern fifty or one hundred years ago and that his professional grandfather may have been further ahead than he himself is right now.

Zusman's work is noteworthy in that he begins by attempting to define consultation but finds that in order to do so, his definition must be so general that it can encompass almost any interaction between a mental health professional and someone who is not a mental health professional. Consultation as it is presently practiced, at least according to Zusman's definition, is not a very distinct area of expertise.

REFERENCE

Caplan, G.: The Theory and Practice of Mental Health Consultation. New York, Basic Books, 1970, p. 144.

Chapter One

THE PRACTICE OF MENTAL HEALTH CONSULTATION: SOME DEFINITIONS FROM SOCIAL THEORY

MURRAY LEVINE

CONTEMPORARY interest in mental health consultation stems from Caplan's (1959) presentation to a conference on social work education in 1955. From a historical viewpoint, it is fitting that Caplan spoke to a social work conference, since consultation was a regular professional activity in the early child guidance clinics. In those clinics, largely staffed by social workers, professional mental health workers acted in consulting roles to teachers, probation workers, visiting teachers, and child welfare workers.

Consulting practice started then for the same practical reasons as now: an inability to provide sufficient direct services to meet public need. Even in the 1920's, it was apparent that any agency attempting to provide a direct therapeutic service would be swamped beyond its means. The child guidance clinics were established in large part to provide a diagnostic and consultative service to other social agencies so that the other agencies might carry out their functions more effectively. From the earliest history of our field, it was apparent that we would never be able to provide direct services, although we lost sight of the fact for a whole variety of reasons we have discussed elsewhere (Levine and Levine, 1970).

PROBLEMS IN THE CONSULTING ROLE

In the past, as in the present, when the urgency of social

problems forced our attention to the issue of how we deliver services to the masses of people, a consulting role was devised and justified on economic and logistical grounds. There are, however, important problems in developing the consulting role on such grounds. It is very doubtful that the logistic problem will be met by such an approach, if our experience at the Psycho-Educational Clinic in working with schools is any guide (Sarason et al., 1966). Imagine a school with six hundred children, 20 per cent of whom are identified by their teachers as having important educational or emotional problems, and having in many instances severe social problems, family disorganization and social agency involvements. Consultants working two to three days a week in such a school barely had time to make the rounds to stay current with fast-moving events in the most difficult cases, much less cover all the classrooms and children.

Part of the problem stems from the makeshift arrangements which place a consultant in a school without a defined role (Newman, 1967; Sarason et al., 1966). When there is no place in the school's organization for the consultant, many problems enter which reduce the consultant's efficiency in making the rounds. Case conferences and group consultations help, but these are limited to after school hours because someone needs to cover the classroom. The situation is clearly difficult in public schools, but similar issues arise in all agencies in which the workers have defined tasks to carry out with no relief available. Prison guards, probation workers, recreation personnel, or welfare workers all have work loads and responsibilities which limit participation. A cottage parent may have time when children are in school, but he usually has other duties during that time; furthermore, all the cottage parents have the same free time. If they are to be seen on an individual basis, it is clear that the amount of prime time available for consulting is really quite small. Those of us who have trained in clinic or social agency settings in which case conferences, seminars, and supervision are built into the structure are continually surprised at the miniscule amount of time devoted in other types of institutions to cooperative planning for case management, or to achieving conceptual clarity concerning the human relations aspects of the work.

The fact that we have to struggle to find the time and place to be consultants is important to note. That fact tells us that what is important to us is not necessarily important to others, and that the workers in settings unfamiliar to us may perceive other aspects of their tasks as critical for them. We will return later to this issue of how the worker's perception of his task affects the consulting relationship.

There are other problems inherent in the consulting role which are obscured by an emphasis on the economical delivery of mental health services. One of these concerns our professionalism, which requires us to look at ourselves as trained practitioners whose technique is applicable across the board. We tend to ignore ourselves as social beings, yet it is we as social beings who must relate to others who are also social beings. We are aware of the difficulties of trained psychotherapists in relating to blue collar, lower class, black and other ethnic minorities. There are differences in values, in styles of communication, in therapeutic goals, in preferred methods, and in expectations about the nature of the doctor-patient relationship which require attention if a working relationship is to be developed at all.

The situation is no different when mental health professionals attempt to relate to the so-called caretakers. It has long been true in medicine, increasingly true in psychology, and probably in psychiatric social work as well that practitioners are coming from upper middle class backgrounds. Teachers, policemen, welfare workers, and similar caretakers tend to come from blue collar and lower middle class backgrounds. If the problems are not approached with due attention to the relevant issues, the consultant will find himself working with the restricted population of caretakers who happen to share his assumptions about the world. Many others will be missed or unnecessarily put off.

An example will clarify the issue. A group of teachers were talking about how to handle profanity among their children. Many alluded to some of the vulgar expressions their children used, but without actually using the vulgar terms. Verbal dashes filled in for the pungent phrase the child had actually used. At one point the consultant asked, "Well, how do you react when a child says, 'Fuck you' "? Rather than elicit discussion, he noted that his free use of the term had resulted in a shocked and embarrassed silence. Discussion brought out the teachers' feelings that such vulgar terms were not meant for polite discussions in mixed company, that the consultant's use of the word had created a great deal of discomfort in several of them. Here was a clear value difference in communication style which had to be respected and understood if the consultant were to continue to work with that group.

A problem related to how we deliver services concerns that which we deliver. It is a truism with important consequences that professionals do what they have been taught to do. Moreover, professionals take pride in and value certain abilities and accomplishments for what they imply about professional skill. A surgeon may convince other surgeons that the operation was a success despite the death of the patient, but it is harder to convince the patient's family. Hughes (1951) points out that nonprofessionals judge performance by the success or failure of the outcome while professionals look to the artistry of the performance itself as an index of success. In other words, those skills which the professional values in the context of the social organization of his typical practice and when he uses other professionals as his reference group, may not be applicable in new settings in work with caretakers.

A classic example is found in David Levy's (1952) discussion of the typical course of consulting relationships between psychiatrists and workers in other agencies in the early days of child guidance. Trained in mental hospitals, in a Kraepelinian tradition in which diagnosis was highly valued, many psychiatrists knew little else. In their consulting relationships, they provided others with the labels of psychopathology. At first, it was reassuring to agency personnel to know they were dealing with a case of dementia praecox or a psychopathic personality, but after awhile, agency personnel would become adept at making their own diagnoses, and would ask for directions about how to maintain the patient in the community. At that point, the limitations of psychiatric knowledge would become painfully apparent, and a degree of disenchantment would set in.

A rather similar cycle ensued when psychiatrists learned and employed the technical language of psychoanalysis. While there was little problem in those agencies which moved toward a casework or a treatment orientation, in many other settings, the nonanalytically oriented personnel soon learned that a knowledge of deep dynamics did not translate into a practical program of management. Sometimes, caretakers were so appalled and put off by the "down, deep and dirty" id-oriented terminology of the psychoanalysis of that day that a relationship could not develop (Ridenour, 1948). Just as diagnosis was not enough, so interpretation of dynamics was, and is, far from sufficient.

A further problem arises when we consider the implications of the fact that the ultimate targets of a consulting practice are not the caretakers, but rather the population under care. It is the urgent demand for the development of solutions to social problems which has rekindled interest in consultation; this means that the target population are members of the underclass. They are the welfare families, the delinquents, the criminals, and the drug addicts. These groups tend toward impulsive, often violent behavior patterns, or they tend to exhibit apathetic and passive-aggressive modes of resistance to intrusions by the institutional representatives with whom mental health consultants ordinarily work.

Few of us in the mental health fields have had much to do with the underclass, either through personal life experience, or in professional training. In our normal practice, we value and select as patients or clients those who share our assumptions, and who will accept the conditions under which we offer help. The various forms of filters we employ in our treatment settings effectively turn down, or "cool out" those who are unwilling to accept our assumptions about the world. What we come to learn are those approaches which are more or less effective in our psychotherapeutic relationships, the social contexts in which we practice therapy. It is a remarkable blind spot in mental health professionals who take on consulting roles that permits us to provide advice to caretakers in dealing with their charges when our own base in experience is with different social groups; and we admit to ourselves that we reach the underclass badly or not at all with our approaches. Typically, we are not faced with dealing with tough, "street smart" people, on a day-by-day basis, and we often compound our innocence by naively viewing the poor as the noble savage, free of the bourgeois vices evident in our colleagues, and present in offensive degree in the upwardly striving caretakers who consult us. If our consulting advice to caretakers is to act toward their charges as we would act toward our patients in our settings, it is not clear that we will be performing a useful service. To advise talking out problems with children who respond only to firm action is not helpful, and may be destructive.

CONSULTATION AND SITUATIONAL THEORIES

Much of what we have said is prelude to the argument that an atheoretical view of consulting practice based on economic and logistic considerations may miss the point. An effective consulting practice requires a theory which takes into account the complexities of the social world in which consultant, caretaker and client all participate. It is crucial to recognize the very obvious, but elementary circumstance that the caretaker, and the subject of his care, our ultimate client, participate in a socially organized enterprise in which both have a stake. The caretaker has a mission to fulfill. If he is a full-time worker, he has an economic stake: retention on the job, avoidance of the displeasure of his superiors, and advancement all depend on the fulfillment of his mission. Moreover, if the caretaker has some identification with his occupation, his sense of personal fulfillment is at stake. At a realistic level, no one can live comfortably and view himself as incompetent in his job, or worse yet, as destructive of the welfare of others. No schoolteacher could continue teaching and believe what some self-styled educational experts and prophets are saying — that teaching destroys the minds of children.

Because caretakers are so intimately involved with doing their jobs, it is a basic assumption of consulting practice that caretakers will define as problems those people who in some way interfere with the caretaker's ability to fulfill his mission, as he perceives his mission. The assumption is critical, for it argues that psychopathology, as mental health professionals understand the term, is not the central issue. Rather, what is important is the interaction of the role of caretaker (with all that implies in the technical meaning of the term) with the role assigned to the client. Complicating the interaction are the personal and idiosyncratic characteristics of the role incumbents. We emphasize the social role concept here, primarily because mental health professionals tend to know the personality issues far better, and in consequence overlook the role issues.

Having said that much regarding role interaction, the statement is still rather empty. We cannot say, given the present state of knowledge, what ought to be determined and weighted. However, such a broad statement is still useful because it forces us to look at issues beyond those to which theories of psychopathology ordinarily call our attention. Most theories of psychopathology, upon which consulting practice tends to depend, are based upon what we have elsewhere called the assumption of intrapsychic supremacy (Sarason et al., 1966; Levine, 1970). We assume that if a person is having a problem in living, that problem is caused by inner needs or other intrapsychic factors which determine his perceptions of his world and the actions he takes in it. Such theories assume a fairly narrow range of normal behavior, and they assume that the pathology causing abnormal behavior is carried around within the individual. Thus, we believe we can assess pathology by examining the individual in a psychiatrist's office, or we can give him psychological tests in the psychologist's office; what is wrong will show no matter where the patient is examined.

Alternative views have been propounded. Assume that the range of behavior which could be exhibited by a healthy, intact person and still be considered normal, is very wide. In such a view, abnormality is a function of societal reactions to unexpected or atypical behavior patterns. In our society, if a man goes into a period of isolation and withdrawal, is depressed, agitated and fearful, apparently hallucinates, or has fits in which he throws himself on the ground writhing and screaming, we define him as sick. We send him to a doctor who provides the complimentary role to the patient role. We incorporate a large variety of rewards and punishments to make it profitable for a man to enter the sick role, and which make it difficult for him to reemerge from that role. We produce a patient, often a chronic patient (Scheff, 1966; Zusman, 1969).

Yet there are other groups in which the same behavior is taken as a sign the individual is very special in another way. When he emerges from his acute distress, he may be given a role as a priest or healer (Kiev, 1964). The definition of the individual as a problem arises when we do not have a defined place for individuals who show unexpected behavior. This model was developed by Scheff (1966) to explain chronic mental illness in the United States. However, the basic tenets of his position that abnormality − or to use his term, "deviance" − is a function of the labeling and subsequent societal response to unexpected behavior, allows us to argue that caretakers are among those who contribute importantly to the definition of behavior as deviant.

We may now revise our earlier stated assumption and assert that caretakers are likely to label as deviant those individuals who exhibit unexpected behaviors* which interfere with the caretaker's ability to fulfill his mission. Note, it may be important to the caretaker to label the individual deviant in order to place the problem behavior outside the accepted range of competency of the caretaker. He can continue to validate his sense of self as a competent worker, despite his failure to accomplish his purposes with that particular individual. As a prison guard, he can control the normal criminal, but not a crazy man who upsets everybody by his loudness and his bizarre attempts to hit his head and fists on a wall.

THE CONSULTANT'S ROLE

Before developing other implications of social theory, it is necessary to discuss the consultant in his role. While a consultant requires highly developed clinical sensitivity and skills, his skills need to be adapted to the problem at hand. From the viewpoint of the caretaker, it is his client who is the problem and probes designed to elicit the caretaker's involvement with the problem person are often viewed as accusations that the caretaker is at fault. After a relationship has developed, and when the consultant and consultee have learned something about each other's implicit

---

*We are using the term unexpected behavior as a synonym for Scheff's term, "residual deviance," in order to save time and space. Consult Scheff for the necessary definitions.

assumptions about the world, it is possible to move more readily into consideration of the details of emotional involvement. However, it is likely that we will not be able to count on the ready acceptance of the idea that a caretaker is always emotionally involved with his client (as we can in psychotherapy supervision), until the mental health professional has had a greater opportunity to influence the basic education of various caretaking groups. A consultant works toward the acceptance of the idea of emotional involvement, but he cannot expect that the caretaker will routinely accept that assumption.

In the context in which he works, it is important to recognize that a consultant can only influence; he has no power. He can suggest, advise, help others to work things out, but he cannot give directions and expect that others will have any obligation to follow his directions. The consultant needs a high tolerance for frustration and a low need to control.

The role of consultant and the role of leader should not be confused. The consulting function, particularly in its teaching and problem-solving aspects might well be carried out by the formal leader in a setting, or by his designates.* Because of that fact, whether or not the formal leadership carries out such a function, a consultant may well be viewed as a competitor of the leadership. If actual control of the setting is not at stake, then the consultant will be viewed as a competitor for the affections and respect of those who work in the setting. This issue is best faced by demonstrations of proper respect for the formal leader. Periodic consultations with various levels of administration is necessary to maintain cooperation and to renew sanction. Consultants will frequently use personal contacts or resources in order to give something special to the leader. A consultant might agree to

---

*It is said the consultant works effectively precisely because he has no evaluative function in the setting. In our work we have seen numerous instances in which a skillful principal can be a very effective consultant to his teachers. Unfortunately there are few principals who define their jobs in this way, few who have the time to do it, and few who have the necessary interpersonal skills. We would suggest that such supervisory and consulting skills ought to be part of the armamentarium of a whole range of supervisors, despite the fact that they also evaluate. Changing the definition of the supervisory role and changing the training of supervisors could have a very salutary effect on many service systems.

accept a diagnostic referral from the leader, for a friend for example. In another setting, a certain amount of cooperation was obtained when the consultant and the leader wrote a report together which placed the leader in a good light with his peers and his superiors. Such tactics may buy cooperation over the short run, but in times of difficulty, the consultant may expect to encounter a "what did you do for me recently" attitude.

The one form of power the consultant does not have, and should not believe he has, is attributed to him. He is assumed to have magical powers. He is assumed to be in command of those incantations, which if properly muttered will result in the immediate and absolute cessation of the problems presented by the problem person. Magical powers are probably always attributed to the witch doctor who is in contact with the spirits. If one accepts the death of God, and His replacement with the deities of science, (or in this day and age, their successors, whatever they may be) one may view the mental health professional in a position analogous to the witch doctor. The role relationship may well tap into some deep archetypal layer of belief. The questions from the consultee: "What should I say to him?" or the frequent response to suggestions, "I tried that and it didn't work" (meaning the suggested mode of response was used once and the problem behavior recurred on another occasion), may be taken as evidence of the wish for magical solutions. Every therapist is aware of the wish for magic in his patients, in their requests for formulations or talismans which will ward off evil automatically and permanently. It is no different when a consultant, faced with a consultee under stress, feels ineffective and helpless in doing a good job, and thereby feels threatened. An excellent magical formula is to assert, "I have no magic."

We must be clear about one more point, and that is whose agent the consultant is. As mental health professionals, our primary goal is to provide a form of service to those who are served by or forced to use certain institutional settings. We work for children in school, clients of the public assistance system, delinquent children on probation, and prisoners in a correctional institution. In that sense we are the agents of the clients of the institution and our primary concern is in promoting their well-being. In many institutional settings, and particularly in those under severe public criticism as ineffective (e.g. schools, public assistance agencies, police), the caretakers, our consultees, are frequently under stress in fulfilling the social tasks assigned to them. We are or should be equally concerned with promoting their well-being. The critical problem arises if we conclude that there would be a major conflict between the interests of the clients and the interests of the consultees, no matter what else was true. If we really believe for example that schools in their present organization and mode of functioning really destroy children — "death at an early age" — then we would have no business helping such an institution to do its work more effectively by supporting the caretakers. Similarly, if the sole purpose of a consulting contact in a prison was to reduce the likelihood of riots or escapes by helping to make the custodial and security arrangements more perfect, and helping to make the inmates become more automatonlike, then we would have no business in the setting. Unless a consultant has some hopes of contributing to changes in the way in which institutions function, he should not spend his time in any setting which is truly destructive of the human spirit.

In most instances, consultants assume that the interests of clients and caretakers are not inherently in conflict. Moreover, consultants tend to assume that the social setting and the caretaker's role are sufficiently flexible so that relatively small modifications in the caretaker's methods of responding will be beneficial to both the caretaker and his client.

If a consultant is to work with a situational theory of the kind advocated here, he needs first to understand the situation in which he is working. In the beginning stages he must spend time becoming familiar with the people, with the organization, with its stated and unstated missions, and with the internal tensions which might exist. He may not fully discover these for a long time, but he needs to be alert to ways in which his role might be shaped, and how he might be drawn into a variety of internal struggles.

As a resource (in several meanings of that term) entering a social situation, the consultant can be viewed by those already present both as advantageous and as threatening. In some settings his attention might be valued because caretakers see him contributing to their prestige. The supervisor of a unit in a residential center welcomed the presence of a consultant because he saw a way to bring himself to the attention of his superiors for a promotion. In elementary schools, predominantly occupied by women, a male consultant may become the object of sexual competition for his favorable attention. In still other situations, a consultant's attention is viewed as threatening because he was brought in to help those who were incompetent to help themselves. A consultant may expect that no matter how he is presented, ambivalence toward him will inevitably be a factor, with all degrees and combinations of positive and negative feelings expressed toward him by different members within the setting (Levine, unpublished manuscript).

INTERVENTION STRATEGIES BASED ON SITUATIONAL THEORY

Using a situational theory, emphasizing the concept of role, we would now like to provide illustrations of three general types of interventions toward which a consultant may strive. The illustrations will be taken largely from our work in schools, but the concepts are general, stemming from the theory that problems are defined in the interaction of the "role" of caretaker and the "role" of client.

The first type of intervention strategy is what might be called relabeling. It will be recalled that the situational theory argues that caretakers label unexpected behavior and respond in terms of the label assigned. In a sense, by labeling behavior as deviant, the caretaker requires the other person to enter the "sick role" or the "bad role." Others, for example the psychologist or the assistant principal, then play their parts as well. If the labeling process can be modified, subsequent actions will also be different.

Teachers of young children commonly complain that the children do not finish their work. The child's difficulty in completing the work is rarely attributed to the length of the assignment (because most of the other children do finish it), or to the boredom of the assignment. Boredom is a term which implies criticism of the teacher. The teacher is rightly concerned about the incompletion of work because she believes the assignment contributes to the child's learning, and because she needs to have tangible evidence the child is learning in order for her to feel she is being a good teacher. The incomplete work may be attributed to "immaturity," a term implying that the child does not belong with his peers; to laziness, implying moral condemnation and a need for punishment; or to excessive daydreaming, implying psychological disturbance and a problem beyond the range of competence of the teacher. In each instance the label provides the ground for action, or inaction.

Before the case is brought to the consultant's attention, the teacher has already attempted solutions based on a label. The consultant's problem is to help the teacher relabel the behavior in such a way that the teacher feels the behavior falls within her range of competence and understanding. She can then take action in relation to the new label. The laziness label may stem from the teacher's feeling that her sense of competence is under attack by the child's apparent unwillingness to do the work. Rarely, however, does the teacher's feeling of anxiety and anger become the focus of attention. More typically, a consultant will sympathize with the teacher's desire to do a good job and to elicit any extraneous sources of anxiety (e.g. an aggressive parent, a fear her class as a whole will not be good enough on achievement tests), and then he will try to develop some alternate interpretation or label for the child's behavior. The child's problem in completing work may be attributed to a desire for perfection, and a fear of making errors — a fear which may be viewed as originating in the child and in the home, and not having its source in the teacher's approach. Under these circumstances, a teacher may come to feel the child is cooperating with her in her teaching function rather than attacking her as a teacher, and she may feel more inclined to provide a form of support for the child (e.g. smaller bits of work, frequent reminders to complete the work, encouragement designed to relieve anxiety).

In previous work (Sarason et al., 1966), we provide a number of examples of how one might change the teacher's perception of a problem. We have since noted that consultants in school settings going as far back as the visiting teachers of the early 1900's

(Levine and Levine, 1970) and the child guidance clinics of the 1920's (Wickman, 1928) have discussed similar tactics. It is helpful if the child's problem can be seen as a reaction to a normal crisis (e.g. reaction to divorce, parental illness, responsibilities to younger siblings) which elicit the teacher's sympathy. It is much more difficult to achieve changed attitudes if the consultant offers a psychodynamic explanation for behavior which is offensive or morally repulsive. To understand all may be to forgive all, but too often the psychodynamic explanation is viewed as an excuse for the behavior. The consultant's dynamic explanation may be viewed as a demand that the behavior be accepted or overlooked, and that the caretaker is wrong or too neurotic to be concerned about it.

Alternatively, an explanation of the behavior as a normal manifestation of childhood which needs to be socialized can be accepted and acted upon constructively. A kindergarten teacher reported that a boy and girl engaged in what was to her obvious sex play, in that the boy mounted the girl and embraced her. She did not know what to do. During discussion with a consultant, she was helped to see the behavior as a natural form in children, and was encouraged to control its more blatant manifestations gently but firmly in the classroom. Once given permission (we shall return to this point below) to control what was in her view disruptive behavior, she was also able to admit to her own discomfort in viewing the behavior in children. The consultant and teacher then engaged in a constructive discussion about sex education for young children. An interpretation of the behavior in oedipal terms, or the consultant's failure to acknowledge the problem of classroom management presented by the sexual behavior might well have disrupted continued contact between teacher and consultant.

The use of diagnostic labels presents some very special problems. Unless there are excellent and accessible facilities for dealing with problems of mental deficiency, brain damage, or emotional disturbance, the provision of such labels may result in the teacher's decision that the problem falls outside her range of competence, and the "hands off" phenomenon sets in. Without direction or support, the teacher may ignore or isolate the child, declining to work with him out of the very understandable fear, promoted in part by mental health professional propaganda, that she might harm the child (Sarason et al., 1966).

The phenomenon of a diagnostic label resulting in "hands off" may be seen in a variety of settings. In a state hospital unit for children, delinquent adolescents were routinely labeled sociopaths, or "acting out," and thereby were viewed as not belonging on the unit for "psychotic" children. The behavior of the psychotic children was more obviously bizarre, and sometimes more dangerous in terms of self-inflicted injury or impulsive injury inflicted on others, but a psychotic belonged and a sociopath did not. Dr. David Reynolds of the Erie County Mental Health Department has called attention to the related problem of overdiagnosing. If a child is labeled as psychotic and retarded, he may be refused acceptance into services which deal with either diagnosis, but not with both. If he accumulates enough diagnostic labels, he may be made ineligible for all institutions and services.

In an employment center a similar problem arose. A diagnosis of simple schizophrenia almost resulted in a refusal of service. The relabeling of the client "as a man who needed a quiet, nonstressful job in which he had minimal contact with other people," led to a position for him. In another instance, the consultant found it necessary to help workers in the center to distinguish between a homosexual and a man who needed a job.

Relabeling is not a matter of verbal trickery. Sometimes the simple act of relabeling will relieve a caretaker's anxiety sufficiently to permit him to act; however, a concerted plan of action still needs to be developed based on the new label. Relabeling requires an ability to translate technical concepts into everyday language. Dr. James Robinson, Director of the Child Psychiatry Clinic at the E. J. Meyer Memorial Hospital, emphasizes that he will relabel in terms of trite everyday slogans, anecdotes and parables or in terms which draw direct analogies to the caretaker's experience. A consultant took it as a sincere compliment when a teacher told him, "You know, it's funny. You don't talk like a college professor."

A second set of intervention tactics may have to do with helping to provide a special role or a special place for the individual who is exhibiting the unexpected and unwanted behavior. Alternatively, one might help to provide rules or conditions under which the unwanted individual becomes socialized and nondisruptive. Teachers normally use such tactics regularly. An attention-seeking child may be provided with the job of being class reporter or secretary, and may read the minutes of the class or call the attention of others to himself in a socially acceptable manner. A child may see himself as more responsible if he is made a line leader, or is provided with a regular job, making him a helper. Several teachers have reported excellent results in changing sullen, aggressive, difficult children into more cooperative and tractable human beings by providing a role as a student teacher and giving the children responsibility for teaching a portion of a lesson. Recent experience has suggested that older children who themselves have academic problems are helped by providing roles for them as tutors for younger children. A teacher provided an "office space" for a child who needed a retreat in his class. Another had a spot which could be used at will when an adolescent needed to sleep during the day. Another had a talking corner where children could converse with each other freely, although there were defined rules for carrying out the activity. The behavior which was previously disruptive became socialized. In the antipoverty program, adolescents much preferred to see themselves as employees of the program, rather than as people who were being helped by the program. The role of employee was more desirable and prestigious than the role of an inadequate person taking help.

A consultant may help a caretaker to use the concept of role in managing problems. A consultant who is new to a setting may have some problem in helping a caretaker to create such solutions because of his unfamiliarity with what is possible. As experience accumulates, the consultant may find that his bag of tricks enlarges as he learns from skillful caretakers in the setting. He then is in a position to help to diffuse innovations which have proven themselves feasible in that setting. It is helpful if the caretakers can teach each other, but then the consultant needs to help manage the competitiveness which may arise between caretakers. The adoption by others of such tactics is complicated when the caretaker feels such special privileges should be used as rewards for otherwise conforming behavior, and not as roles which will stimulate desirable forms of expression. The caretaker's imagination and patience set further limits. However, as regards disruptive behavior, a consultant may help a caretaker to see that he spends a considerable amount of time with the disruptive individual anyway, but not in a time and form of the caretaker's choosing.

The third form of intervention focuses more directly on the caretaker's role. The limits of a role — "what is my job and what isn't" — are often ambiguous, and are often defined by different role occupants in quite different ways. In many settings, caretakers encounter certain problems because of the way a role is defined. The role may be defined too narrowly, or the caretaker may place unreasonable demands on himself.

Often a caretaker already has good ideas about how to handle the client's problem, or a relatively brief discussion elicits a working plan. If the consultant asks why the plan was not already implemented, he is often given the reply that the principal, or the supervisor or the "office" would not stand for it. Sometimes the caretaker's judgment is correct, but equally often the restriction in action comes about because of a narrow definition of what is permissible within the role. For example, as simple a matter as programming for a child who cannot read at grade level is viewed as a difficulty because the teacher believes that she is not allowed to use a book which does not belong in that grade level. In some of our schools, we found that teachers rarely made home visits themselves although many expressed a wish to do so, and that there was no rule against home visits. Encouragement by a consultant resulted in some home visits. Another teacher seemed to need permission from a consultant to fuss over a little boy, straighten his tie, help him to wash his face or brush his hair back in motherly fashion, because she believed a teacher was not supposed to touch a child. In these instances, the consultant provided what we have called authoritative support (Sarason et al., 1966), and what others have called "giving permission" for teachers and principals to do what they feel needs to be done. The consultant uses his interviewing skills to help the caretaker arrive at a possible solution, and then encourages the caretaker to go ahead and do it. It sometimes takes permission from someone with at least the cast of authority to have the caretaker extend the repertoire of behaviors encompassed within the role.

The role and person sometimes intermingle in more complex ways. Young teachers in high school settings sometimes find themselves treated as sexual objects, or they find themselves attracted to students as sexual objects. The sexual attraction can create role failure as a teacher, conflict for the teacher, or can result in defensive distance from interaction with students. Young teachers will sometimes feel ashamed of their feelings or confused by them. Authoritative support can help.

A young teacher reported terrible discomfort in the halls because boys would whistle at her or make remarks to her. She felt flustered, and would feel embarrassed and blushing whenever it would happen. Discussion revealed she experienced the problem as difficult because such things were not supposed to happen to a teacher. When the consultant asked how she would handle the situation as a girl, she had half a dozen answers. The next time she reported she had stunned the group of boys with a girl-type of put-down, and reported feeling relieved that she had mastered the problem.

All new teachers, and many more experienced ones, need to learn to master techniques for maintaining discipline. The problem is compounded by the inevitable inadequacies of teacher preparation. But many young teachers, themselves barely through an adolescent rebellion, have grave difficulty in accepting the authority role and in accepting adult responsibility as a teacher. Moreover, the young teacher frequently experiences helplessness and rage when children do not obey. Many will turn against themselves for feeling and acting toward their children as all their hated teachers did. Distinct problems in accepting the authority role, and distinct problems in coming to terms with one's feelings of anger interact with conceptions of what is appropriate to the teacher's role. Severe problems in managing an entire class can result, although the problem is usually accentuated by the presence of one or more provocative and difficult-to-handle children in the class.

A consultant sometimes can help a teacher work her way

through the conflict, and become more firm and demanding of the children without feeling hostile to them. Sometimes the strain is so great that all are better off if the teacher seeks another more congenial assignment. In such situations, a consultant is on familiar grounds, for he can respond to teachers who open up the issues with him much as he would in a therapy situation. Where the teacher is more defensive and less inclined to self-exploration, the consultant may be limited to a more sympathetic and supportive role, if not for the sake of the children, then in support of the teacher as a human being in distress.

Many of the problems are extraordinarily difficult, and are insoluble without additional resources. A consultant needs to be careful that he does not add to the burden of guilt by implying that the problem could have been solved by a more capable caretaker. A consultant may be better advised to work to reduce the self-imposed demand that the caretaker must handle all aspects of the problem even though the resources are not available.

The sight of a neglected child in a school stimulates feelings of pity and a need to do something about the situation. A teacher can, within limits, provide for the child during the school day, or may go beyond the call of duty and provide clothing for a child, or even take him home on weekends. Nonetheless, the basic responsibility for the child remains with the parent and society at large. A single teacher cannot be expected to fulfill all that a stable home would provide. It sometimes becomes the consultant's duty to help the caretaker accept such limitations without excessive guilt. The consultant can help to spell out what can and cannot be reasonably accomplished, and can use the authority and respect attributed to him to help the role incumbent modify the concept of the role.

The caretaker's role may have some built-in problems which arise because of the way in which the caretaker's work is organized, beyond anything the caretaker as an individual contributes. The teacher's job in most public schools is organized so that a classroom teacher is isolated from adult contact. Placed in a room with twenty-five or so very different children, the teacher with one personality and a necessarily limited repertoire of modes of relating to others, is assumed to be equally effective with all of the children in the room. If a child is not learning, that situation is rarely viewed by the teacher as a consequence of an accidental mismatch between child and teacher. At some level, the teacher views the child's failure to learn as her failure to teach. The teaching task itself has a regressive pull, in that the teacher is required to pitch communications at a level suitable to her charges, and to identify with them in order to understand and communicate. The teacher is not looking forward, but going over ground she herself has previously mastered. As any parent will attest, the degree of affect aroused when dealing with children can be very great, but schools seem to assume that affect is irrelevant to the task of the school. Not only are there few channels within which affect can be discharged, but the isolation is compounded by the implicit assumption of school organization that to ask for help is an admission of failure. Teachers are not told to expect problems or to come for help routinely. Rather they are told, "Come for help only when you cannot handle the problem." Beyond its isolation, the task of teaching is draining. Few other occupations require so much continual giving and provide so few indices and recognition of successful achievement as teaching. The social organization of teaching provides little by way of nutriment to replace the emotional energy which is demanded and consumed in the day-by-day work of teaching.

Because schools are organized in this way, one of the primary functions the mental health consultant fulfills is that of providing support and encouragement. The consultant can help provide nutriment for a caretaker who is doing a good job, and who in the normal course of events gets little replenishment. In such a social context, the consultant's approval, his words of praise, his general support and his attitude of sharing in the problem provides something which is lacking in the setting. It is no small contribution for a consultant to use himself to replenish that which a skillful and dedicated teacher provides for a difficult and demanding child. In effect, the consultant becomes a part of the total social system by adding a resource it lacks. He helps the system to maintain itself and to function at a higher level of effectiveness.

Consultants sometimes feel such a role is difficult to fulfill, because it is quite undemanding of any exercise of skill on the part of the consultant. Supporting the very skillful efforts of others, particularly when the consultant has real doubts as to whether he could perform nearly as adequately as his consultee, and when he knows his rate of remuneration is much above that of the consultee, may produce anxious moments and guilt feelings in the consultant. On the other hand, the support would be less meaningful if it came from a peer, or from a person of low prestige. It is, in part, the consultant's social position which enables him to be effective in the setting, and given American culture, it may be necessary to accept that bit of irrationality and to use it effectively.

THE FUTURE OF CONSULTATION

Having developed a view of consulting practice grounded in social theory, it is also necessary to assert that consulting practice itself is probably the least important aspect of the consulting role. There is already evidence piling up that consultative interventions do not lead to enduring changes (Byrne et al., 1968; Cowen et al., 1966; Pierce-Jones et al., 1968) in a clinical sense. However, the advantage of the role as a research device should not be underestimated. When the consultant is able to work in the caretaker's setting, he gains a much more intimate knowledge and awareness of situational determinants of problems in living. He becomes much more aware of the totality of forces surrounding every human issue. We have already become aware that there are more and better ways of dealing with the deviant than defining such individuals as outside the pale, and isolating them. Beyond the problem of dealing with deviance, however, is the problem of the design of helping services so that the human tasks can truly be carried out. The consulting role will enable the mental health professional to come to understand the social nature of human interaction. Based on previous experience, it may be both predicted and fervently desired that mental health professionals will turn their attention to the problem of the design, in a social sense, of those institutions in which we live our lives, so that the institutions support a full life.

REFERENCES

1. Byrne, R. H., et al.: The Elementary School Project. Final Report, University of Maryland Research Center of the Interprofessional Commission on Pupil Personnel Services, 1968.
2. Caplan, G.: Concepts of Mental Health and Consultation. Washington, D. C., Childrens Bureau, 1959.
3. Cowen, E. L., et al.: Prevention of emotional disorders in the school setting. J Consult Psychol, 30:381-387 (Oct), 1966.
4. Hughes, E. C.: Mistakes at work. Canad J Economics Political Sci, 17:322-325 (Aug), 1951.
5. Kiev, A. (Ed.): Magic, Faith and Healing. New York, Free Press, 1964.
6. Levine, M.: Some postulates of community psychology practice. In Kaplan, F., and Sarason, S. B. (Eds.): Collected Papers of the Psycho-Educational Clinic. Springfield, Mass., Massachusetts Department of Mental Health, 1970.
7. Levine, M.: Problems of Entry in Light of Some Postulates of Practice in Community Psychology, unpublished manuscript.
8. Levine, M., and Levine, A.: A Social History of Helping Services: Clinic, Court, School and Community. New York, Appleton, 1970.
9. Levy, D. M.: Critical evaluation of the present state of child psychiatry. Am J Psychiatry, 108:481-494 (Jan), 1952.
10. Newman, R. G.: Psychological Consultation in the Schools: A Catalyst for Learning. New York, Basic Books, 1967.
11. Pierce-Jones, J., Iscoe, I., and Cunningham, G.: Child Behavior Consultation in Elementary Schools: A Demonstration and Research Program. Austin, University of Texas, Personnel Services Research Center, 1968.
12. Ridenour, N.: Mental health education. In Lowrey, L. G., and Sloane, V. (Eds.): Orthopsychiatry, 1923-1948: Retrospect and Prospect. New York, American Orthopsychiatric Association, 1948.
13. Sarason, S. B., et al.: Psychology in Community Settings. New York, Wiley, 1966.
14. Scheff, T. S.: Being Mentally Ill. New York, Aldine, 1966.
15. Wickman, E. K.: Children's Behavior and Teacher's Attitudes. New York, Commonwealth Fund Division of Publications, 1928.
16. Zusman, J.: Sociology and mental illness. In Kiev, A. (Ed.): Social Psychiatry. New York, Science House, 1969, Vol. I.

Chapter Two

MENTAL HEALTH CONSULTATION:
SOME THEORY AND PRACTICE

JACK ZUSMAN

CONSULTATION, like psychotherapy, is a word which is loosely defined and used in many ways. Here we are going to focus on mental health consultation.

Mental health consultation is the process in which one person, by mutual agreement defined as a mental health expert, formally undertakes professionally to advise another, called the consultee, regarding individuals for whom the latter has responsibility to provide help. The consultee is usually employed by a "helping agency," that is, one which assists persons who are having problems in living; the agency is not considered to be within the mental health service system. The mental health service system means the collection of agencies and practitioners who see themselves and are seen by the public as dealing with problems of mental illness or involuntary interpersonal maladjustment.

It is apparent that even this attempt to define the field leaves our subject very poorly delineated. Each of the terms in the definition needs further consideration. For example, it is paradoxical, but it seems true, that mental health in the term "mental health service system" means something different from mental health in the term "mental health expert." In the latter case, mental health is much more broadly defined so that the mental health expert who serves as the consultant is expert in problems of mental illness and interpersonal maladjustment — yes, but also in the areas of human development, normal interpersonal relations, behavioral science, and often in the applications of social and behavioral science. Mental health consultants work in many kinds of agencies where their functions are very general and go far beyond the scope of mental health service agencies which usually deal with the mentally ill and disturbed. Perhaps it would be clearer if we talked of mental illness agencies or mental illness service systems in contrast to mental health consultants. However, this is not done.

To pursue the definition a bit further, to advise, which is what the mental health consultant does, means that he suggests a course of action. However, he does not accept responsibility for the outcome and leaves it to someone else to put his advice into practice. That someone else, the consultee, is free to accept or reject the advice. It is the consultee and his agency who take responsibility for the outcome of the problem.

All those working in the consultation field owe much to Gerald Caplan, who among other things has proposed the terms consultee-centered and case-centered consultation (Caplan, 1964). Consultee-centered and case-centered mental health consultants focus on problems which are encountered in working with agency clients. Unlike Caplan, I make no distinction between case-centered and consultee-centered consultation. In practice, I find there often is little difference. A consultation request always arises partly from needs of the client and partly from needs of the consultee. The consultant's response always is partly aimed for the client and partly for the consultee. Although depending upon the situation, the principal focus changes from case to case and a well-trained consultant is able to vary his approach, the consultee usually is not aware of any change in the consultant's focus and is concerned mainly with the client's problem.

Occasionally, the consultant may spend time doing formal education or other activities not directly related to consultation, but his primary function is to advise about particular cases. (This process must be distinguished from administrative or organizational consultation where the consultant makes an effort to produce change in the organization or agency itself. He is employed to deal with agency problems and usually does not concern himself with individual cases. This kind of consultation has been extensively dealt with by others (Bennis et al., 1969) and is only indirectly related to mental health consultation.)

From the vagueness of the definition of mental health

consultation, it should be no surprise that those who work as consultants are often not sure exactly what they are doing. To put it another way, we have very little theory to help clarify our roles and our long-term objectives when we undertake consultation. It is difficult to tell others what to do as consultants. Consultation is presently an art, not a science, and is probably best taught by observation and imitation rather than instruction. This represents a serious weakness, and one purpose of this paper is to present the beginnings of the theory which guides my own work and which I hope will be used as the basis for discussion by others. Without a theory, which is in effect a statement of what we are trying to do and why, it is almost impossible for us to measure whether or not we are having any effect. At present, we often are reduced to following the precept, "If it feels right and everybody is happy with it, then do it."

It has been said that mental health consultation is the central skill of the community psychiatrist (Downing, 1965). It is the most important means through which he carries his philosophy into the community and has an impact many times greater than if he attempted to do any form of direct treatment. From the mental health professional's point of view, consultation may be the only hope for ever reducing the demand for mental health services and thus cutting down the tremendous disparity between supply and demand.

From the consultee agency's point of view, consultation is desirable in that it leads to improvement in staff skills and helps the agency to provide better service for its clients. Not to be neglected is the prestige factor. An agency which has mental health consultation is one up on an agency which does not. For these and a number of lesser reasons, consultation has become an important activity and significant sums of money and amounts of professional time are being spent to employ mental health consultants.

It is distressing, but true, as far as I know, that the value of mental health consultation has never been demonstrated. For those active in the field, it remains an act of faith that we are doing some good and that we ought to expand our activities. Let me hasten to add that the evidence for the effectiveness of mental health consultation is certainly as good as the evidence for the effectiveness of most forms of psychotherapy. Most activities of mental health professionals fall in the same unfortunate category as articles of faith.

One of the ways of looking at consultation is as a transactional process. Consultation is a series of interactions among a circle of people, each of whom is having a simultaneous effect upon all of the others. Consultation in this sense is a system where A not only affects B but B affects A and together they affect C and D who in turn affect them (Fig. 2-1).

In the usual agency practice of consultation, there are four parties and four major relationships. There are the client, the worker or consultee, the consultant or mental health expert, and the worker's supervisor. The major relationships are between client and worker, worker and supervisor, and worker and consultant. In

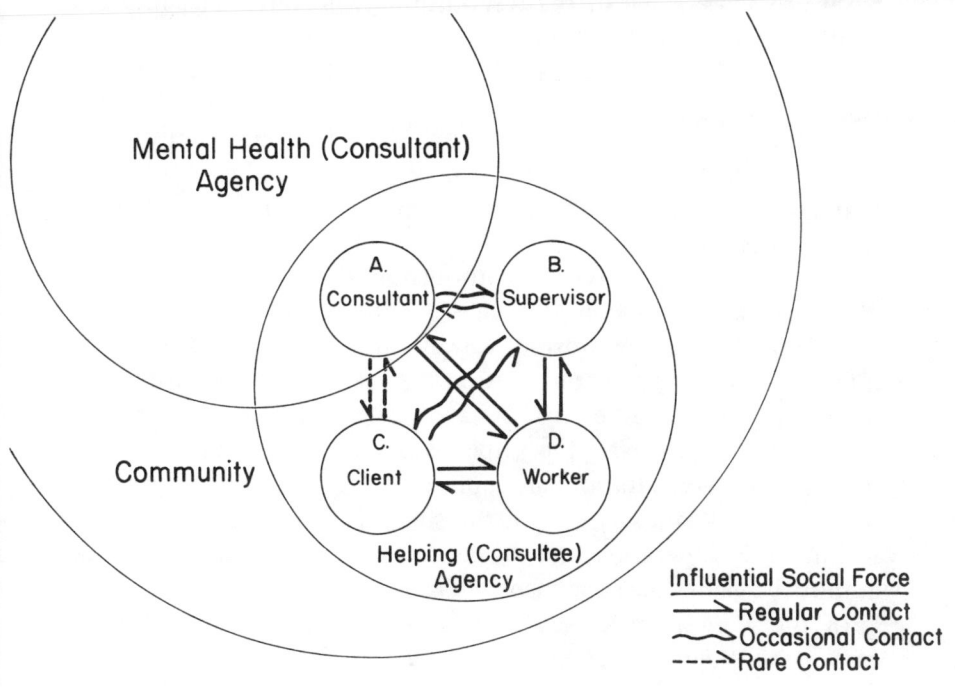

Figure 2-1

some cases, there are also lesser relationships between client and consultant and supervisor and consultant.

The decision to call in a consultant on a particular case is based on distress or concern resulting from any number of factors occurring in one or more of these relationships. For example, in the client-to-worker relationship, there may be a disruption of either the role of the client or of the worker. The client may not respond to the worker's direction, either explicit or implied. The client may become too close and personal or may destroy the worker's image of omnipotence. The worker may lose his "professional armor" and unexpectedly find his personal feelings toward the client to be overwhelming.

The worker may wish to have the weight of the consultant's authority to back suggestions to the client which the worker believes will otherwise be disregarded. The worker may feel the client's prognosis is so poor or his behavior is so frustrating that he wishes to share some of the responsibility, hostility, or guilt with another person and yet may not be able to do this with his supervisor. He may recognize some element in the client which frightens him, such as mental illness or uncontrolled hostility. He may then wish the help of a more skilled or more prestigious person to deal with this. Or, he may wish to abdicate responsibility for the client and may want someone to whom he can turn the case over.

In the worker-supervisor relationship, the supervisor may be concerned about the competence or mental health of a worker. He may also be feeling hostile toward the worker and may be interested in using the consultation as a punishment or a method of forcing the worker to behave. The worker may request consultation to please the supervisor since he recognizes that requests for consultation are important to the supervisor. The worker may also disagree with the supervisor or be feeling hostile toward the supervisor and hope to use the consultant as an authority against the supervisor.

In the worker-consultant relationship, there are also a number of possible themes. The worker may wish to use the consultant to obtain a psychiatric diagnosis or psychotherapy for himself. He may express his hostility to the consultant by picking cases with which the consultant is obviously not competent or in which the consultant's advice is doomed to fail. He may fear the consultant and hope to please or appease him by presenting inappropriately simple cases. The worker may also be looking for someone on whom he can lean and may have the fantasy that the consultant has some magic that will solve all of his problems with the client. Finally, he may simply desire to relate to the consultant. Therefore, he may pick out cases which he is quite able to handle on his own but which will give him something to talk to the consultant about.

The supervisor-consultant interaction may emphasize the supervisor's desire to please the consultant and to encourage him to continue his consultant work with the agency. For this reason, the supervisor may pressure his workers to find cases when there are none appropriate or when there is no interest in consultation among the workers.

When the consultant sits down with the consultee, he has to be aware that many of these themes, as well as others not mentioned here, will be present simultaneously to different degrees. The consultant has to ask himself for what reasons is this case being presented today. He must not assume the reason for presentation is simply the worker's need for information or his recognition that the case requires mental health consultation.

The consultant's response to the worker's presentation is most effective if he answers the implicit questions in the consultation request. To do this, he must use his clinical skills to estimate what the consultee is really asking. When the consultant misjudges the hidden questions, he may step into a trap which someone has inadvertently set for him or he may lead the consultee astray. One of the things which makes consultation so hard is that the consultant usually dare not be so bold as to ask what the real reason for presentation is. Even if he does ask, the consultee is often not fully aware of the reason.

In doing consultation, there are always at least two sets of objectives to be kept in mind. The consultant has one set of objectives and the consultee another. Often, at the beginning of the consultation relationship, these two sets are completely different and very far apart. As the relationship proceeds, the two parties come to be aware of each other's objectives either through explicit discussion or implicitly through their responses to each other. Obviously, if their objectives continue to be far apart and if their actions are in line with their objectives, the two parties will not long remain together. Therefore, in most consultation relationships, as the relationship matures, the objectives on both sides change and begin to overlap. Although even after a long period of time they may never come to coincide, in a good relationship there is a significant overlap. There also is an understanding of each other's objectives to the point where each is willing to tolerate those differences which continue to exist.

The objectives of the consultee are easier to describe. In this case, consultee means the consultee agency rather than the individual worker whose interests we have already discussed. The agency wants more effective service for its clients. In the belief that a mental health consultant can help to bring this about, it engages the consultant. More specifically, the agency usually expects that the consultant will provide some education for its staff, some diagnosis and treatment for its clients or patients, and will help make more effective referrals. These are very obvious objectives. There is a whole group of less obvious but no less important objectives. Some of these are obtaining the prestige of having a mental health consultant; the magical expectation that the consultant will somehow help the agency to solve problems which have been beyond its capability in the past; the addition of a resource to whom it is possible to pass the buck, or at least to use in relieving the agency of responsibility and guilt when a case goes bad; and sometimes the hope that a touch of psychotherapy will be provided for agency staff, particularly for those who have trouble getting along with their supervisors.

Very commonly, the theme which runs through the specific elements of the agency's objectives is desire for direct service. The agency wants the consultant to come in and do something to the clients. The agency wants to see immediate evidence of the consultant's effectiveness.

The consultant's objectives are more complex. Often he is interested in improving the consultee agency. He may want to make it a better source of mental health and mental health related services or just to make it a better community agency. He sees himself helping the workers to do a better job. If the consultant is associated with a mental health agency which provides direct services, he may have the objective of cutting down referrals to his agency by helping workers deal with clients who have mental health problems instead of making referrals. The consultant's agency in fact may be glad to pay his salary and send him out, hoping that by providing indirect service he will reduce the need for a great deal of direct service. His presence may also be a way in which a mental health agency demonstrates its interest in the community and perhaps diverts some of the community dissatisfaction over the limited amount of direct mental health service available.

Not to be neglected in listing objectives are the personal satisfactions which the consultant looks for in the consultation process. There is the gratification from being powerful and respected by a group of workers in another agency. There is also the opportunity to learn about the ins and outs of a whole new care system and to expose himself and his ideas to a new kind of setting.

Last, but by no means least, are the complicated objectives of prevention of mental illness, improvement of mental health, and early diagnosis and treatment. The consultant goes out into the community and into other agencies in the interests of fostering primary and secondary prevention.

If one examines the literature regarding consultation and the literature regarding prevention, it seems clear that despite the hopes of many, there has not been a great deal demonstrated as to how mental illness can be prevented by mental health consultants. We do know very definitely that by treating syphilis early, by preventing children from eating paint containing lead, and by bringing children up in families rather than in institutions, we can prevent serious mental troubles later on. However, these are general principles easily taught in professional schools and a consultant is not needed to carry these messages.

The consultant can carry out secondary prevention – that is, prevention of untreated long-term illness – through helping workers to recognize signs of mental illness and then helping to arrange for immediate referrals. If a case is presented to the consultant and it strikes him that the client is mentally ill, he can point this out to the worker. This is certainly a worthwhile service, yet it tends to defeat one of the objectives which consultants often have; that is, to cut down on the number of referrals.

The consultant can provide information for the consultee to pass on to the client which may be useful in preventing mental illness. For example, if the case involves a mother sharing the bed of a teen-age son, the consultant can point out the problems which this is likely to cause. However, here again, most consultees learn this kind of information in professional schools. In fact, many clients already have a basic minimum of facts concerning what is necessary for healthy development; when things go wrong, it seems to be due less often to ignorance and more often to something else.

This something else needs to concern the consultant a great deal. Certainly, unconscious factors have a great influence on the behavior of clients, and Caplan points out what ought to be obvious — these factors also influence consultees (Caplan, 1970, p. 144). Caplan talks about the theme interference which prevents a worker from relating to a client in the manner for which the worker has been trained and in which he is quite capable with another sort of client. Anyone who has done consultation has seen a number of cases where a competent worker is doing a terrible job and the theme interference stands out. Our problem is how can we do something about these cases and, if we are successful, are we having any effect on the prevention of mental illness and the promotion of mental health?

I have serious doubts with regard to both of these questions. In the average-size agency, the consultant encounters the same consultee usually no more than three or four times a year. Often, the case presented on each one of these occasions is completely different in character from the one presented by the same worker on the previous occasion. Therefore, the same theme interference does not arise and the consultant has the opportunity to do something about a particular theme interference just once.

Since theme interference usually results from unconscious, change-resistant factors, the very limited opportunity to deal with it is discouraging. It does seem that on rare occasions it is possible to produce behavioral and attitudinal change through a single consultation session, provided the consultee is properly primed. The consultee must be extremely uncomfortable with the current situation, have a good deal of preparation for another way to do and think about things and be basically flexible. In such a situation, the consultant provides the slight push which is necessary so that the consultee falls into a new way of doing things.

Although studies of the impact of consultation on theme interference are lacking, we are now coming to recognize that psychotherapy can be effective after no more than two or three or four sessions (Redlich and Freedman, 1966). However, brief psychotherapy works best with people in crisis, people extremely uncomfortable with their situation, and people who are highly motivated to find some way out. In dealing with theme interference, we are not providing psychotherapy but we certainly are providing something which is closely related. However, the consultee's crisis is almost always miniscule compared to that of the brief psychotherapy patient.

I suggest, then, that no matter how skillful the consultant, he usually will not have enough of an opportunity to be effective in changing the consultee to the point where theme interference is eliminated or significantly reduced.

Although I am not hopeful that most single consultation sessions have a significant carry-over to the consultee's work with future clients, I believe a single consultation session can have a profound effect on the life of a single client. Particularly when the client is young, the carry-over may be very long-term and very important.

What I am concerned with is a form of prevention of disability that has been talked about for some time in relation to mental health agencies but has not been extended much to activities in other agencies and other kinds of helping systems. The disability I am referring to involves labeling a person as ill, deviant, or dependent, and the effect this has on the way he sees himself and the way he is seen by others. The clearest cases, of course, come from mental hospitalization. A good deal has been written about patient role and the difference between behavior necessary to be a good patient and to be a healthy person. Many authors have pointed out that in adjusting to the hospital and becoming a good patient, an individual must take on new habits and give up old ones with the result that he may be completely disabled for life as a normal person (Zusman, 1967). Built into most helping systems and institutions is a pernicious force which can injure those being helped. By accepting a client for service, any social welfare agency can cause a good deal of harm, particularly if labels are freely applied or strict conformity to agency customs is unwisely demanded.

The cases where there is incongruity between what a social welfare agency sees as desirable client behavior and what the client actually does, are the ones which are likely to come to the attention of the consultant. It is with these cases that the consultant can be very effective in preventing long-term disability by preventing the agency from inappropriately forcing the client into the mold which the agency provides. In such a battle between agency and client, the client often is forced to choose between giving up the agency's help (which he may desperately need), or taking on the client behavior, which although desirable to the agency, may rob the client of some of his strengths and attachments to independent life.

The consultant's job here is to step outside the agency's system and help the worker-consultee examine which of the demands the agency is making are necessary for solution of the client's problem and which are a part of the traditional response of the agency but serve no essential purpose.

Often, all that is necessary is for the consultant to provide information or to point out to the consultee something which was missed because of the consultee's involvement within the system. In my experience, theme interference resulting from unconscious motivation is not a prominent difficulty in these cases, and so it is easy for the consultee to see the point. Once he is helped to look outside the limits of the system, he and the consultant together can often find a new way of dealing with the problem. The consultee's anxiety about a client who refuses to fit the agency's expectations can often be simply and significantly lessened. This reduction of concern in the consultee and of pressure on the client is one of the very important and very effective preventive functions of the consultant.

The consultant serves a number of other functions which at first glance seem less important and yet which can be very helpful to the consultee. In the day-to-day practice of a busy agency, it often happens that a case is not reviewed from start to finish except when it is presented to the consultant. Sometimes, too, a case is not presented to the worker's supervisor except in preparation for the consultation or at the time of the consultation. Other cases, although previously reviewed, have not been dealt with. Either because of the difficulty or the complexity of the solution, the necessary steps have been postponed.

The presentation to the consultant provides the opportunity for omissions and delays to become obvious. In such a case, the consultation is useful even though the consultant does not provide any knowledge or does not even say a word. His presence has served to encourage the agency administration to examine what it has been doing and to recognize that further steps are needed.

I have heard it said that when such simple cases are presented to the consultant, both his and the agency's time is being wasted. To me, this is not so. The case review was needed and it resulted in action. The action probably never would have taken place except that the consultant was there. I regard this kind of consultation as just as important and as useful as the ones which require the highly developed skills of a very competent consultant. However, perhaps these cases serve as an argument for the use of less skilled consultants on many cases.

If consultation is effective, in what ways does it work? There seem to be a number of reasons why consultation might be expected to work and a number of different mechanisms through which it operates. One of the most important is through the information and advice which the consultant provides. When the consultee's problem stems from lack of information or lack of experience, this may be all that is needed. When future cases of the same type appear, the consultee is better prepared as a result of his previous learning.

As has been previously discussed, the consultant may make a

contribution to the solution of the problem by acting as an audience and providing the occasion for a complete review of the agency's activities and plans with a particular client. In such cases, when the worker and supervisor have the opportunity to do a complete review, the solution to the problem becomes obvious to them. There is not likely to be a carry-over to future cases although the consultee may have learned that it often is useful simply to sit down and examine a case from beginning to end.

The consultant may provide the consultee with the opportunity to ventilate his feelings regarding a difficult case and in this way enable the consultee to return to the problem somewhat refreshed or possibly with a new attitude. The sympathy which the consultant may express for the consultee may also relieve some of the hostility which the consultee feels toward a difficult client. The consultee may feel that some of the responsibility for the case has now been assumed by the consultant, and this may free the consultee to act more flexibly or more vigorously with a difficult client.

The consultant can serve as a role model for the consultee. Just as the client presents the consultee with a problem which must be dealt with, the consultee presents the consultant with a problem. The consultee can observe the interaction and the manner in which the consultant reacts to the problem. It seems quite likely that to a certain extent, the consultee identifies with the consultant. When the consultee next faces the client, he is likely to imitate the consultant as he deals with the client. If the consultant is a good role model and if the consultee is successful in handling the problem, his behavior will be reinforced and there should be a significant carry-over.

Another important function for the consultant is as a facilitator of communications. As the case is reviewed for a consultant, it often becomes clear to him that there has been a breakdown in communication either within the agency or between the agency and some other important organizations. He can identify for the consultee the difficulty in communication, and sometimes can even act himself to clear the channels of communication. Within the agency, he can occasionally make use of his position outside of the hierarchy to establish communication between the two levels which are blocked by bureaucratic structure. Establishment of such communication channels may carry over so that work with future cases is simplified.

The consultant can occasionally be effective as an authority figure, directing that certain approaches be used, rather than acting only as adviser. Indeed, it is all too easy for him to take this role or for the consultee to place him in it. Although in urgent cases this can be effective in producing immediate action, it has long-term drawbacks which are obvious. In addition, it has very poor carry-over to other cases.

A final way in which the consultant is effective is as an intelligent person who is willing and able to use common sense. It often surprises me when a consultee is stumped by problems which do not require any technical expertise but which can be solved by knowledge acquired through the experiences of having lived in a family and worked in a bureaucracy for a number of years. On occasion, the consultee may have a limited experience in an area where the client has difficulties and in which the consultant, as an older and more mature person, is knowledgeable. For example, despite a good deal of technical training, the consultee who is single and has never reared children is likely to have serious gaps in knowledge when advising a client who is having difficulties with child-rearing. In such a case, the consultant may be able to help merely on the basis of his experience as a parent and not because of his special mental health knowledge. At other times, when the client's problem is very difficult and beyond the skills of anyone in the agency as well as beyond the consultant, the consultant merely provides another head for a problem-solving session.

The ethics of consultation is an important and often neglected area. Obviously, the consultant is bound to keep confidential what he learns in his agency relationship. It is not so obvious, however, what his responsibility is if a worker reveals something in confidence which the supervisor would need to know. If the consultant informs the supervisor, he runs the risk of having his consultee, as well as all other workers in the agency, resent him and cut off communication with him. If he does not inform the supervisor and the supervisor learns that he knew, he runs the danger of rupturing his relationship with the supervisor. The consultant clearly does not have a doctor-patient relationship with the consultee, but in the absence of any explicit understanding, there may be confusion about what the ground rules are. Perhaps this is best handled by making an explicit agreement in the beginning of the consultation relationship as to what mutual expectations will be. It may also be handled by having the supervisor present at all consultation sessions.

What is the consultant's responsibility to and for the client? When the consultant is a psychiatrist who is consulting with nonpsychiatrists, it may seem as if the consultant is legally taking on a supervisory medical responsibility. At least, he alone is the physician, and to the layman, and perhaps to the lawyer, has legal responsibility for what occurs. Yet the consultant sees himself only as an advisor and takes no responsibility. This is made more complicated if the consultant sees the client directly on one or more occasions. Usually, these sessions will be for diagnosis, but even so, the question is then raised as to what kind of medical responsibility the consultant may have.

The issue can also arise that the consultant feels the consultee or the agency is not doing an adequate job for an individual client. What should he do then? Obviously, he will work with the agency to improve the service which it provides the client. However, if he feels that good service in this case is beyond the capability of the agency, should he advise the agency to refer the client elsewhere? Should he advise the client to go elsewhere? In either case, he runs the danger of rupturing his relationship with the agency, thus stopping his efforts to improve the situation. I do not know what the answers to these questions are, but I believe these are things which consultants and consultees should be thinking of.

Another important ethical area is the issue of the so-called "hidden agenda." This refers to the consultant's objective to deal with the consultee's theme interference — the unconscious block to effective action. In my experience, the consultant usually does not make clear to the consultee that he is searching for theme interference and that he will attempt to deal with it. To talk about this might interfere with the consultant-consultee relationship and would prevent elimination of theme interference. The consultant proceeds without telling the consultee what he is attempting. The consultee is likely to assume that the consultant is being completely open with him. Yet, this is not completely true. Here again, I do not know the answer but feel the need for more discussion of the issues.

I would like to end with some consideration of the future of consultation. In what direction are we moving and where should we be years from now? Should our long-term goal be to put ourselves out of business? Will we ever be able to eliminate all areas of theme interference and all areas of professional ignorance and eventually eliminate the need for consultation? I would answer possibly, Yes. It seems to me that our objective ought to be to train supervisors to deal with theme interference and to incorporate many of the consultant's insights into professional education programs, thus eliminating the need for consultation. The need for consultation highlights a gap in professional education. Professional educators ought to be studying the experiences of consultants to see where education has failed and consultation has to step in. With a modification in professional training, gaps for which consultation is now required ought to be filled. It is quite possible, however, that with changing living and working circumstances, new areas will evolve where professional education lags. It will be some period of time then before education catches up; in the interim, consultation must take up the slack. By the time education does catch up, there may perhaps be still other areas. As long as society is changing, there may be a need for a consultant to intervene where education has not yet responded. The consultant's essential role may be as a "plugger" of educational and emotional gaps in professional training.

REFERENCES

1. Bennis, W. G., Benne, K. D., and Chin, R.: The Planning of Change, 2nd ed. New York, Holt, 1969.
2. Caplan, G.: Principles of Preventive Psychiatry. New York, Basic Books, 1964.
3. Caplan, G.: The Theory and Practice of Mental Health Consultation. New York, Basic Books, 1970.
4. Downing, J.: Personal communication, 1965.

5. Redlich, F., and Freedman, D.: The Theory and Practice of Psychiatry. New York, Basic Books, 1966, pp. 280-281.
6. Zusman, J.: Some explanations of the changing appearance of psychotic patients. In Gruenberg, E. M. (Ed.): Evaluating the Effectiveness of Community Mental Health Services. New York, Mental Health Materials Center, 1967.

SECTION II
The Consultation Process

INTRODUCTION

THE course of consultation is rarely smooth or straight. Consultation involves the interaction and (it is to be hoped) collaboration of a number of individuals with diverse backgrounds and interests. Looking over the shoulder of each individual is usually an agency with its own history and interests. The agencies themselves are composed of individuals who also have diverse experiences and interests. Thus, consultation is influenced by a multiplicity of prior experiences, prejudices, professional backgrounds, traditions, limitations on resources, and demands. The successful outcome of a consultation process involves exploring all of these factors either covertly or, less commonly, overtly, negotiating the conflicts, compromising, and arriving at some agreement which meets enough of the demands of all of the agencies and individuals involved so that the consultation process becomes worthwhile for them to pursue. In some cases, some of these diverse factors must be neglected or disguised, lest they become so disruptive, particularly at the early stages of consultation, that the whole process falls apart. In such cases it is only later, when relationships have been strengthened by the development of mutual respect and some common experiences, that these emotion-laden issues can begin to be examined and negotiated.

Since a consultation "contract" almost always is not a written contract but rather an informal agreement to work together, the consultation process is maintained only by the interest of the parties involved. At any time, the relationship may be broken off by the decision of one or more of the parties that it is not worth the trouble it entails. Indeed, many consultation relationships have been broken off. Even if not broken off, some consultation relationships degenerate to the point where they result in wasted time, decreased efficiency by the consultee and his agency, and sometimes permanent discouragement, both on the part of the consultee and the consultant. This can happen when goals and interests are in conflict to a significant extent between consultee and consultant, but not quite to the point where the relationship is disrupted. Thus a crippled relationship results which is just positive enough for the partners so that they are reluctant to end it completely but yet not positive enough so that it is really helpful or so that enough interest is generated to produce some progress in developing the relationship.

In his chapter, Graziano, a clinical psychologist who has specialized in developing services for exceptional children, describes the checkered career of one consultant. This consultant began in one role with one set of interests and attempted to mesh with the interests of a group of parents in a community. As the relationship developed, there were problems which resulted in the evolution of the consultant's job into another role. The consultant went from role to role until he reached the final role of unemployed mental health professional. One of the implicit messages of this story and one which is borne out by many other consultation experiences is the strength of the hopes and unspoken demands which consultees and consultants place upon each other. This often occurs despite explicit agreements reached by both parties which may be in contrast to the unspoken elements. Yet, in the long run the unspoken and unsatisfied elements may be the ones which prevail and result in a loss of the relationship.

Rae-Grant, a psychiatrist with extensive experience in administering a community mental health service, discusses in his chapter some of the errors which consultants commonly make. Many of these errors are ones which result naturally from a background as a mental health professional, and particularly a background of extensive training in psychotherapy. Many of Rae-Grant's points serve as examples of the general maxim that unspoken expectations carried over from previous situations often are inappropriate and disruptive. What will work very well in a psychotherapy situation with a patient who expects treatment will not work at all in a consultation situation with a professional who expects to be treated as a colleague. Although both Graziano and

Rae-Grant emphasize the negative, they do so in order to draw quite clearly the outlines of the positive.

Chapter Three

THE CONSULTANT, THE CLIENT AND HIDDEN ASSUMPTIONS

ANTHONY M. GRAZIANO

CONTRACTS AND RENEGOTIATIONS

ONE important point in consultation work involves the need for negotiation of a contract between consultant and client, and the dangers involved in changing roles without clearly renegotiating the contract. In one of my first consulting experiences, I verbally contracted with an agency to provide certain psychological services to develop a therapeutic program for children. In a short time, because of the growth of the agency, I became a supervisor rather than a consultant; shortly after that, my role was restructured and I became a program director. The agency grew rapidly and in a short time my role again changed and I became director of the entire agency. Shortly after that, we again restructured and I became, sadly, unemployed.

The process required some four years to complete, during which time there was rapid change in the agency. The consultant was the major change agent and led it to develop in directions which markedly differed from what was later defined as the original intent of the agency. The major difficulty was the lack of a clear definition of the agency's goals and the consultant's role. As a result, the two parties proceeded along their own divergent assumptions, unaware of the differences which led them in opposed directions while assuming they were in agreement. The agency or client and the consultant failed to specify their goals, to perceive the differences between their respective sets of assumptions or to recognize that the rapidly changing nature of the agency required careful and frequent reevaluation and clarification of tasks and roles, i.e. to continually examine the consultant-client relationship.

In this specific situation, the agency and the consultant held different assumptions, different sets of expectations concerning the nature of the task at hand. We were in apparent agreement: the task was to develop effective services for children. However, we also held hidden assumptions which eventually emerged in strong conflict. These hidden assumptions, briefly, were as follows: the agency's board of directors, all nonprofessionals, assumed that the consultant, a trained professional, would have the necessary skills, "all the answers," so to speak, so as to develop and maintain "treatment" programs for their children.

On the other hand, I, as the consultant, did not share that assumption. My assumption was that I had skills which could create and maintain an ongoing therapy program. However, since the field had had such little success with severely disturbed children, I also assumed that any stable program could be only a minimum, a "point of departure," a base for further work. The crucial task, then, was to continue both an intensive inquiry into the behavior of the children, and a constant upgrading and change process of the basic program.

My model was one of seeking effectiveness through continual change; the board of directors' model was one of finding the "right program," and then keeping it going with little change needed.

The conflict was inevitable. In two years, the program had developed to a smoothly functioning, apparently highly successful therapy program. The children seemed to be benefiting and even casual observers noted the greater order, cooperation and increasingly "normal" behavior of these heretofore bizarrely behaving children. The program included not only specific programs for children, but also direct work with parents, staff recruitment and training, and even provided some services for other agencies. Thus, as the laymen saw it, the major goal — direct services for their children — had been achieved. Except for some expansion in the number of children and the eventual acquisition of better facilities to house the program, they were quite satisfied with the level and quality reached. The program, they believed, was a complete, "finished" program, henceforth requiring primarily only maintenance. They were puzzled, then, when I continued to modify what appeared to be an already adequate program. The consultant believed we had achieved only a minimum stability necessary to continue the important work of continued inquiry, evaluation, and program improvement.

Because the assumptions were unverbalized, each party believed the other shared his own assumptions. Therefore, their behavior was mutually inexplicable. The laymen did not understand why, since they apparently agreed on program goals, the psychologist continued to change the apparently complete and well-functioning program; on the other hand, the psychologist could not understand why, again since they apparently agreed on goals, the laymen continued to block progress and resist the changes which were necessary to achieve the program goals.

Unrecognized and unverbalized, these basic differences persisted and after another two years, despite the operation of an excellent program, the agency disintegrated.

THE CONSULTANT AND THE CLIENT'S VALUE SYSTEM

The second incident I wish to describe is a more recent example: How does the client perceive the consultant, and how do such perceptions affect the nature of their working relationship? As the following example should make clear, a consultant ought to know a good deal about the client's values. I recently accepted a consulting task in a large, maximum-security state prison which housed some two thousand long-term felons. I had agreed to develop a token economy program in a cell block of eight men, as part of a larger rehabilitation project. A basic requirement for success of the token economy was to obtain the active cooperation and support of the men housed in the cell block. Accordingly, I met with them individually and in small groups, getting their reactions, suggestions and criticisms, and their collective pledge to support the program. After several months of discussion, I became ill and had to remain at home for three consecutive weeks. The prison was informed that I would be absent for a period of time, but the prison authorities did not explain my absence to the prisoners. During those next three weeks an interesting development took place. As I failed to appear, my prestige among the prisoners increased. By the time three weeks had elapsed many of the prisoners were referring to me with words of great respect, praise, and esteem, clearly indicating that they had developed an extremely high evaluation of me during my three-week absence. This high level of evaluation, however, plunged sharply immediately upon my return the fourth week. In fact, there was a noticeably negative tone to the prisoners' greetings to me when I returned.

Why? What had happened to create such sharp increase in esteem and why should it abruptly end immediately upon my return? Let's look at the situation from the prisoners' point of view. They saw a stranger with the title, "doctor," introduced as having certain skills, who moved in, "talked up" and developed a good deal of enthusiasm for his particular project. They had heard rumors of a federal grant totaling from fifty to one hundred thousand dollars, contingent upon the consultant's ability to persuade state and federal officials that he offered a project worthy of such support. Within a few weeks they heard that the money had been granted and was "on its way." Shortly after that, just when the money was expected at any moment, the consultant disappeared, and no more was heard of a project or of fifty or a hundred thousand dollars. One week went by, two weeks, and then three. By then, the prisoners put together an explanation based on the available facts and rumors, and congruent with their own value system which elevated the consultant to the high-status level of a "super con-artist" who was convincing that he "conned" the "cons" themselves, as well as the state and Federal Government. By this time, they thought, he was away in a southern French resort or some other plush place, living it up with the one hundred thousand dollars. "By God," they mused admiringly, "he did it!"

Upon my return to the prison project, banal reality intruded and my status plummeted. I was, after all, nothing more than a "straight" psychologist representing "straight" society, merely doing his job and being, in reality, no different from any other "cop," regardless of profession. It required another two weeks to overcome enough of their disappointment to work easily again with them.

SUPERVISION: SELECTION OF NONTRADITIONAL PERSONNEL IN MENTAL HEALTH AND EDUCATION

In the remainder of this paper I would like to discuss briefly my experiences with one of the possible tasks in a consultant's role, i.e. the selection of nontraditional personnel. Although the task included selection, training, and supervision, I would like to focus here specifically on the selection process.

It is frequently asserted that one of the major reasons for the scarcity of mental health services is the lack of sufficient manpower. It is argued that the professional schools do not train enough therapists to provide the services needed. This argument is based on the assumption that services "needed" can be provided only, or perhaps best, by "trained therapists" who graduate from professional schools. In recent years, the assumption that only professionals can intervene in cases of emotional disorder has been questioned and even rejected. What is "psychotherapeutic" does not necessarily occur only in "psychotherapy" or by ministration of a highly trained psychotherapists. One of the recommendations of the Joint Committee on Mental Illness and Health (1961) included this point. They stated:

> Every effort must be made, then, to provide non-psychiatrically trained personnel in many fields with as much knowledge of mental illness and principles of its treatment as possible. They are treating the mentally and emotionally disturbed and will continue to do so. They must be given additional skill [p. 123].

Attempts to implement this suggestion have been reported by Holzberg (1963), and Knapp and Holzberg (1964), who noted success with college student volunteers in "Companion" and "Aide" programs for state mental hospitals. Branch (1963) wrote of the need to develop new kinds of mental health personnel and Rioch et al. (1963), reported a successful program in training married women as psychotherapy "technicians." Goodman (1964) described attempts to create a training program for nurses to improve their understanding of mental illness and its treatment, while Schurmans (1965) and Armstrong and Rouslin (1963) indicated that the nurse can be qualified to do intensive group psychotherapy. Christman (1966) described a neighborhood day treatment program for posthospital mental patients in which indigenous, nonprofessionals were trained and employed in casework, rehabilitation and family services.

The work thus far mentioned attempted to train nonprofessionals to provide variants of traditional psychotherapeutic service. An even greater departure has occurred during the past decade, as behavior modification concepts have led to training nontraditional personnel in equally nontraditional services, such as behavior modification. For example, training ward personnel in behavioral approaches to modify even grossly bizarre behavior has been reported by several writers. Ayllon (1963, 1967), and Ayllon and Michael (1959) discussed the significance of training ward personnel as "behavioral engineers" and thus affecting significant improvements in patients. Blackwood et al. (1969) described their successful modification of bizarre behavior of severely retarded adults. In one demonstration, they trained ward personnel in the use of positive and negative reinforcers in order to control patients' behavior which consisted of frequent, daily vomiting by one patient who would then be joined by the others in eating the vomitus. Whitney and Barnard (1966) discussed the use of operant training methods by ward personnel to improve the self-help behavior of severely retarded patients.

Bachrach et al. (1965) report the treatment of a thirty-seven-year-old woman who had decreased in weight from 118 to 47 pounds. The experimenters used a variety of reinforcers, applied by ward staff, to increase her eating. They enlisted the aid of her family to generalize and maintain the new, adaptive behavior.

There has also been a considerable amount of work with children, in which significant adults, including parents, have assumed therapeutic duties. Wolf et al. (1964) trained attendants and parents to apply laboratory methods to alter serious behavioral handicaps in an autistic child. Davison (1964) discussed a program for training college students in social learning therapy with autistic children. Graziano (1963, 1967, 1969a), and Graziano and Kean (1967) reported their use of subprofessional group workers in group behavior modification programs with autistic children. Browning (1967) utilized treatment center staff as social reinforcers in a behavior modification program which successfully reduced stuttering in a schizophrenic child.

Wetzel (1966) reduced compulsive stealing in a ten-year-old boy by using nonprofessional persons such as one of the institution's cooks, in the observation, recording, and contingency management of the boy's behavior.

Patterson and Brodsky (1966) utilized parents, teachers, peer groups, and experimenters as treatment agents in modifying hyperaggressive, fearful, and negativistic behavior in a five-year-old.

In addition to many other demonstrations of the use of nonprofessionals in actual therapeutic roles, there have been discussions of the implications of these "new therapists" in terms of the type and availability of services and training of new personnel (Graziano et al., 1967; Poser, 1967; Graziano, 1963, 1967, 1969, 1969a).

In education, too, nonprofessional or "auxiliary" personnel have filled a variety of roles for many years, and are being employed in increasing numbers. The National Commission on Teacher Education and Professional Standards (1967) estimated that ten thousand aides were working in proverty projects alone, and predicted that the number will grow to several hundred thousand in a few years. The New York State Education Department (1966) found that 428 of the 629 school districts surveyed were employing a total of 3,134 teacher aides. The National Education Association (1967) reported an estimated 400,000 man-hours of assistance to elementary teacher aides in 217 school systems surveyed.

The use of nonprofessional aides in schools has been focused primarily on easing the burdens of the teachers by assuming the more routine, noncreative tasks. Some writers, however, such as Klebaner (1967), and Levine and Graziano (1972) assert that the nonprofessional can be employed in even more important and creative ways. Klebaner, for example, contends that the nonprofessional teacher aide perceives himself ". . . as someone helping children, not [as] someone doing the things teachers do not like to do [p. 13]." In this vein, nonprofessional aides have been increasingly employed in more meaningful duties which entail direct involvement with children. Several writers, such as Bayles

(1967), Karowe (1967) and Shipp (1967), argue that a major contribution of nonprofessional aides is the increased staff-to-student ratio which would provide greater opportunity for adult-child interactions. These writers believe that such increases in contact and presumably in communication and influence would be particularly valuable for helping economically disadvantaged children. With reference to that population, Kobrin (1965) discussed the use of indigenous volunteers in delinquency-prevention programs, and Pope and Crump (1965) give "case examples" of the employment of school dropouts to assist teachers in preschool programs.

In many of the projects described in the literature, the nonprofessionals, volunteers or paid, were often mothers of the school children. Mothers have been used to improve health services in schools (Hawkins, 1967); to assist in teaching emotionally disturbed children in special classes (Donahue and Reing, 1966); as substitute teachers in regular classes (Bracket, 1967; Craymer, 1968); and to conduct reading programs in both regular and remedial classes (Thomas, 1967; Cunningham, 1967).

One of the few reports of a systematic attempt to employ mothers to aid in teaching their own children is that by Hayman and Johnson (1963). The mothers were active in home programs to teach a foreign language to their elementary school children.

In 1963, however, when we began our program, there was little in the literature about non-professionals assuming active and responsible therapeutic and educational roles for severely disturbed children. Likewise there was little experimentation with the active involvement of parents in carrying out special educational or therapeutic programs for their own children.

In 1963, I had become involved in the development of day care treatment and educational programs for psychotic and other severely disturbed children. During the first four years of these programs, sixty-one staff positions were created and filled, all with nonprofessional personnel; I would like to describe the process whereby we selected those people. The conceptual basis of the programs was a behavior modification model. That is, we had suspended psychodynamic concepts, based on our conclusion that psychodynamic therapy has failed, in more than fifty years, to clearly prove its usefulness with psychotic children. Over the next four years we developed a consistent and systematic behavioral approach to the treatment and education of severely disturbed children. One of our basic assumptions was that because behavioral approaches are parsimonious, straightforward techniques, they can be readily taught to nonprofessionals. One of our initial tasks, then, was to locate and train a sufficient number, which eventually totalled fifty-three persons who were nonprofessional or at least "nontraditional" personnel. The selection of new nonprofessionals as trainees was carried out in a subjective but quite careful manner, and included three ways of locating potential trainees: (1) direct appeal to the public through newspaper advertisements, (2) posted notices at two colleges and (3) a standing request for referrals with several colleagues. By far the most effective was the direct newspaper advertisement, and I would like to describe it.

On one recruiting occasion there were seventy-seven replies to the following newspaper advertisement: "Mature dependable women with one or more years of college, nurse's training, or nursery school teaching, wanted to train for work with young, exceptional children. Preference given to applicants with grown children."

By requiring some college experience we presumably increased the probability of attracting applicants with at least average intelligence. Our preference for applicants with grown children was based on the perhaps doubtful assumption that people who have successfully coped with the task of raising their own children would be more mature, patient and knowledgeable than those who had not. Despite the indication of preference for "mature" persons, there was a wide range of applicants from young, unmarried girls to young mothers with teen-agers, and several quite elderly persons, including one great-grandmother.

Each of the seventy-seven applicants was then contacted by telephone, and based on those conversations, thirty-four were eliminated for some of the following reasons: three had already taken other jobs; nine had wanted less than half-day positions; one refused to be designated as only a "trainee"; three expected to work for only one or two months; two had not known what "exceptional children" meant, and were not interested in working with emotionally disturbed children; four would have transportation problems coming from suburbs to center city each day; one was afraid of "that section" of town; and eleven refused to work for such low wages.

The remaining forty-three were then invited to attend a meeting where they would be told more about the position and after which they could fill out application forms. Four persons did not appear, leaving thirty-nine who attended the meeting. The women were told more about the children and their behavior, the kind of work carried out, and the demands made upon the staff. High demands, long hours and low pay were stressed, as well as the potential compensations of seeing severely disturbed children slowly improve. Questions were asked, answered, and a general discussion was carried out, after which those still interested were invited to fill out an application form and choose one of the indicated times for a personal interview. Four, all of them elderly, did not fill out an application, believing the work would prove too physically demanding for them, and three younger women also left because the job was not what they wanted. Thus there remained thirty-two serious applicants for one position, all willing to work for low wages, and all meeting at least the minimum requirements set forth in the newspaper notice.

Thirty-two personal interviews were held, during which further screening of applicants was attempted. The criteria used were subjective and admittedly vague, clearly reflecting not only an attempt to assess rationally the desired characteristics of a good child therapist, but also our own personal biases. In these interviews a total impression of the applicant was sought, arrived at through carefully made qualitative judgments.

Thus, as each applicant was interviewed, very subjective criteria were used to search for a person who was intelligent enough to understand and learn concepts as well as applied techniques, who could easily verbalize his own ideas and who was capable of preparing daily notes and other reports. The potential therapist had to be personally flexible, easily able to accept and to learn ideas conflicting with his own. He had to be able to tolerate uncertainty, to accept unexpected events. He had to be mature, and a dependable person who was capable of good judgment, steady performance, and highly responsible behavior. There also had to be a "quiet calmness" a "softness" about this person, a "gentleness" of approach but coupled always with firm, unruffled maintenance of limits. He had to enjoy working with children, to find satisfaction in noting even small steps in minor progress, to engage in the many instances of gentle humor as well as the more demanding aspects of the work.

In short, the most basic general characteristic deemed necessary is a genuine humanitarian concern for, and a deep enjoyment of children. The personal characteristics sought in a very personalized subjective manner included intelligence, kindness, maturity, flexibility, calm gentleness and firmness of application, an enjoyment of children, a gentle humor and a genuine, deep humanitarianism, all in an essentially action-oriented person.

Several "extremes" were quickly rejected: (1) the overly intellectualized, highly efficient and somewhat "grim" people, rejected because they might become so task-oriented as to lose sight of the "humanness" of the children; (2) the "gushing," overbearing, "all-giving mother" overflowing with limitless "love" for children, rejected because the effect of such people might be to perpetuate infantile and dependent behavior in the children; (3) the previously trained psychodynamic specialist who automatically thought in terms of interpreting inner psychodynamics. The latter were rejected because they appeared so inflexibly sure of their knowledge that, rather than contributing to the development of new ideas and approaches, they were more apt to superimpose the traditional and generally irrelevant psychodynamic framework.

One might object that the persons sought could not be found, not only because the criteria are subjective, and the selection process highly personal and idiosyncratic, but also because the criteria appear to be impossibly demanding. We contend, however, that within the limits of our ability to make such subjective judgments, an abundance of such persons can be quite readily found in the general population. There are probably more than enough persons with the requisite personal characteristics to provide services for all children, of whatever disorder. Our subsequent experiences tend to support that contention.

Based on those thirty-two individual interviews, another ten persons were eliminated because of physical and age limitations, apparent immaturity, unwillingness to commit themselves to more than a few months, rigid adherence to psychodynamic theory, and apparent high anxiety and reactivity. The remaining twenty-two were called in for another interview with me, and then a third, in which they were interviewed by the chief group worker, who had been selected more than a year earlier by a similar process. The group worker was asked to judge the applicant's potential not only for working with children, but for cooperating well with other staff. The group worker and I then independently ranked the applicants and found exact agreement on the top-ranked eight persons and the bottom-ranked four. We agreed that any of the top-ranked eight applicants would probably do very well as trainees, but that the first three seemed to have even exceptional potential. Accordingly, we invited the first-ranked person, a youthful grandmother who had completed two years of college many years ago and who had never held a full-time job before, to accept the position. It was explained that the first two months would be only a trial period, and we had agreed that it could be ended during that time by mutual consent, initiated by either of us. She accepted the position and continued in the various programs for four years, when she moved to another state because of a business transfer for her husband. The second- and third-ranked applicants were hired later when more positions became available.

During the four years of operation of this program, sixty-one positions became available. As seen in Table 3-I, fifteen of the positions were in the "Regular" program which ran from September to June, and forty-six were made available during the four summer camp seasons. Eight persons were invited to return to work each summer and thus the total of sixty-one positions were filled by fifty-three different persons. Table 3-I also indicates the "occupational areas" from which these staff members were selected.

As seen in Table 3-II, the 357 persons who made application learned of the program through a variety of avenues, from newspaper classified advertisements and bulletin-board notices at

TABLE 3-I
PROGRAM STAFF AND OCCUPATIONAL AREAS
FROM WHICH THEY WERE DRAWN

Previous Occupations	Regular Program	Summer Program Only	Totals
Housewives (no college degree)	6	–	6
Nurses	2	–	2
Teachers	1	15	16
College students	6	17	23
High school students	–	6	6
Totals:			
No. of staff	15	38	53
No. of positions	15	46	61
No. of applicants	171	186	357

TABLE 3-II
AVENUES OF FIRST CONTACT WITH APPLICANTS

Avenue	Regular Program		Summer Only	
	Applied	Hired	Applied	Hired
Personal invitation	2	2	–	–
Newspaper ad	140	4	–	–
University notices	19	4	114	17
Recommended by poverty agency	3	1	33	6
Recommended by educational colleagues	5	2	35	15
Recommended by mental health colleague	2	2	4	–
Totals	171	15	186	38

colleges, to personal invitations by the program director. Of the fifty-three persons hired, fifty-one were selected through interviews, much as described earlier. The remaining two were not carefully interviewed and screened, but had been hired early in the program on the recommendation of a colleague in the mental health professions. It is interesting to note that one of these two resigned within two weeks and the other was later discharged for poor work.

Six of the fifty-three persons hired were high school students from poverty homes, hired on a special summer project, and were not intended to be considered "therapists," "teachers," or "group workers." Their responsibilities in the program were clearly limited.

The remaining forty-six staff members, composed of housewives, nurses, teachers, and college students had greater responsibilities, and constitute a group we suggest as potential, nontraditional mental health personnel.

Thus far, the selection process and criteria, and the behavior desired of the therapist has been described. Based on these admittedly qualitative and personal criteria, forty-six persons were hired as trainees to work directly with emotionally disturbed children, and seven high school students were hired as aides with limited duties. Once hired, however, how well did these people perform?

One person resigned and two others were discharged for unacceptable work. Another four, all hired during the brief summer program, had difficulty handling the children and showed so little improvement during the course of the summer program that they would not be rehired nor recommended for further work with emotionally disturbed children.

There was a good deal of variation in performance among the remaining forty, from a minimum acceptable performance all the way to exceptionally fine, consistent work. There were several nontraditional persons whom I would have no hesitation in favorably comparing with any psychiatrists, psychologists, or social workers in terms of their ability to carry out psychotherapy with children. Such judgments are qualitative, but are based on a great deal of careful observation. Thus, forty of these nontraditional staff were judged to be competent, reliable persons who can effectively work as therapists in mental health programs for children. All, of course, would continue to need professional supervision, but many could function with only a minimum of supervision. This is particularly true of those who had worked in the program for two years. Table 3-III summarizes this information.

There is no doubt that an abundance of interested persons did

TABLE 3-III
SUMMARY OF INFORMATION ON NONTRADITIONAL STAFF
(Not Including Six High School Students)

Original Occupation	*No. Accepted*	*Would Be Recommended Again*	*Would Not Be Recommended Again*
Housewife	6	6	–
Nurse	2	2	–
Teacher	16	12	4
College student	23	20	3*
Totals	47	40	7

*The three college students who would not be again recommended were all education majors planning to become teachers. Thus, the seven persons who would not be recommended to work with children were teachers or future teachers!

exist and there were many more applicants than positions available. Based on our experiences, we conclude that locating applicants for positions in mental health programs is a relatively simple task posing no problems beyond the careful investment of time in reaching beyond traditional sources. This appears particularly true during the summer when a vast pool of teachers, college, and high school students are available for as long as three consecutive months of full-time work. If that pool were to be utilized, there would probably be ample manpower to staff all of the mental health summer programs needed for children. Further, the teachers, housewives, and college students trained during the summer could continue to be utilized throughout the entire year, even if on a part-time basis, thus maintaining many of the expanded programs of the summer.

During the four years, it became apparent that when selection is carried out with care, albeit qualitatively, potentially good child therapists can be identified in the general population and, their lack of professional background notwithstanding, trained in relatively short time. We believe that this city is not significantly different from others and thus are convinced that any city can yield a sufficient number of potentially effective child therapists to provide services for all of its exceptional children!

To find and train these people requires a shift away from traditional professionalism, and calls for the exercise of infinite care in both selection and training, essentially still a subjective process of judgments. The current dearth of child therapists in all areas seems due not to any real lack of persons with required talent, but, rather to the severely limiting self-defensive reactions of mental health professionalism. Thus we maintain and stress that potentially effective child psychotherapists exist in abundance in any city, and can be readily identified and trained if we, as professionals, are flexible enough to seek, identify and accept them. The mental health professionalism may have imposed artificial limitations on the supply of child therapists, but this situation need not continue, particularly if we are more concerned with the progresss of children than with the perpetuation of mental health professionalism.

THE CONSULTANT, THE CLIENT, AND HIDDEN ASSUMPTIONS

The three experiences described above all illustrate the same point — clients and consultants must be aware of and examine their own and each other's assumptions regarding their common tasks. As illustrated by the first two incidents, unquestioned and unspoken assumptions held by clients and consultants can easily conflict and create difficulties, sometimes great enough to destroy the consulting situation. It appears particularly important, then, for consultants initially to specify their "contract" as clearly as possible. Perhaps the consultant, because of his professional status, bears the major responsibility of carefully examining and questioning his own and the clients' assumptions.

In the third example, examining and questioning traditionally held assumptions led to widening the role of the consultant to the more active one of supervisor and to developing useful alternatives to traditional staffing and training approaches.

In summary, then, in any consulting situation, the client and consultant should carefully examine not only the obvious tasks and expectations, but also their more subtle, usually unvoiced, assumptions. Further, as they continue their association, many aspects of the tasks may change, requiring reexamination, reclarification, and renegotiation of their agreement.

REFERENCES

1. Armstrong, S., and Rouslin, S.: Group Psychotherapy in Nursing Practice. New York, Macmillan, 1963.
2. Ayllon, T.: Intensive treatment of psychotic behavior by stimulus satiation and food reinforcement. Behav Res Ther, 1:53-61 (May), 1963.
3. Ayllon, T.: Training Non-professionals as Behavior Therapists. Paper presented at American Psychological Association, Washington, D. C., 1967.
4. Ayllon, T., and Michael, J.: The psychiatric nurse as behavioral engineer. J Exp Anal Behav, 2:323-334 (Oct), 1959.
5. Bachrach, A. J., Erwin, W. J., and Mohr, J. P.: The control of eating behavior in an anorexic by operant conditioning techniques. In Ullmann, L. P., and Krasner, L. (Eds.): Case Studies in Behavior Modification. New York, Holt, 1965, pp. 153-163.
6. Bayles, B. C.: New branches grow on the educational family tree. Nat Elem Principal, 6:16-17 (May), 1967.
7. Blackwood, R. O., et al.: Modifying social behaviors in severely retarded patients. In Graziano, A. M. (Ed.): Behavior Therapy with Children. New York, Aldine-Atherton, in press, 1969.
8. Bracket, P. C.: Substitute training at Belmont. Nat Elem Principal, 6:18-22 (May), 1967.
9. Branch, C. H.: Preparedness for progress. Am Psychol, 18:581-588 (July), 1963.
10. Browning, R. M.: Behavior therapy for stuttering in a schizophrenic child. Behav Res Ther, 5:27-35 (Feb), 1967.
11. Christman, J. J.: Group methods in training and practice: Nonprofessional mental health personnel in a deprived community. J Orthopsychiatry, 36:410-419 (April), 1966.
12. Craymer, H. S.: Hart day: Parents take over so teachers can attend a guidance conference. Instructor, 77:47 (March), 1968.
13. Cunningham, M. W.: Corrected reading program using volunteer help. Catholic School J, 67:70-71 (March), 1967.
14. Davison, G. C.: A social learning therapy programme with an autistic child. Behav Res Ther, 2:149-159 (Sept), 1964.
15. Donahue, G. T., and Reing, V. A.: Teacher-moms help emotionally disturbed pupils. Nation's Schools, 78:50-52 (Sept), 1966.
16. Goodman, C.: Implementing Public Law 182. Nurs Outlook, 12:59-60 (Jan), 1964.
17. Graziano, A. M.: A Description of the NOMIC Day-Care, Treatment Program for Autistic Children: A Behavior Modification Approach.

Mimeographed working paper, 1963.

18. Graziano, A. M.: Programmed Psychotherapy: A Behavioral Approach to Psychotic Children. Paper read at Eastern Psychological Association, Boston, April, 1967.
19. Graziano, A. M.: Clinical innovation and the mental health power structure. Am Psychol, 24:10-18 (No. 1), 1969.
20. Graziano, A. M.: Mental health, psychotherapy and the new psychotherapist. J Psychiatr Nurs, 7:69-72 (March-April), 1969a.
21. Graziano, A. M., and Kean, J. E.: Programmed Relaxation and Reciprocal Inhibition with Psychotic Children. Paper read at American Psychological Association, Washington, D. C., 1967.
22. Graziano, A. M., et al.: Training Behavior Therapists. Symposium held at American Psychological Association, Washington, D. C., September, 1967.
23. Hawkins, W.: Volunteers in the school health program. Nat Elem Principal, 46:29-30 (May), 1967.
24. Hayman, J. L., and Johnson, J. T.: Parents help educate their children through instructional television. J Exp Educ, 32:175-178 (Winter), 1963.
25. Holzberg, J.: The companion program: Implementing the manpower recommendations of the Joint Commission on Mental Illness and Health. Am Psychol, 18:224-226 (April), 1963.
26. Joint Commission on Mental Illness and Health: Action for Mental Health — Final Report. New York, Basic Books, 1961.
27. Karowe, H. E.: How volunteers can help disadvantaged children. Children, 14:151-155 (July), 1967.
28. Klebaner, R. P.: School volunteers, a new challenge. Nat Elem Principal, 6:13-17 (May), 1967.
29. Knapp, R. H., and Holzberg, J.: Characteristics of college students volunteering for service to mental patients. J Consult Psychol, 28:82-85 (Feb), 1964.
30. Kobrin, S.: Values and problems in the use of the indigenous volunteer in delinquency prevention programs. In 100,000 Hours a Week: Volunteers in Service to Youth and Families. New York, National Federation of Settlements and Neighborhood Centers, 1965.
31. Levine, M., and Graziano, A. M.: Mental health intervention in the elementary school. In Golann, S., and Eisdorfer, C. (Eds.): Handbook of Mental Health. New York, Appleton, in press, 1972.
32. National Commission on Teacher Education and Professional Standards: Auxiliary personnel. Nat Elem Principal, 46:6-12 (May), 1967.
33. National Education Association: Teacher Aides in Large School Systems. Education Research Service Circular No. 2, The Association, Washington, D.C., 1967.
34. New York State Education Department: Survey of public school teacher aides. The Department, 1966.
35. Patterson, G. R., and Brodsky, G. A.: A behavior modification program

for a child with multiple problem behavior. J Child Psychol Psychiatry, 7:277-296 (Nos. 3-4), 1966.

36. Pope, L., and Crump, R.: School drop-outs as assistant teachers. Young Children, 21:13-23 (No. 1), 1965.

37. Poser, E. G.: Training behavior therapists. Behav Res Ther, 5:37-41 (Feb), 1967.

38. Rioch, M. J., et al.: National Institute of Mental Health pilot study in training mental health counselors. Am J Orthopsychiatry, 33:678-689 (July), 1963.

39. Schurmans, M. J.: Five functions of the group therapists. Am J Nurs, 64:108-109 (Dec), 1964.

40. Shipp, M. D.: Teacher aides: A survey. Nat Elem Principal, 6:30-33 (May), 1967.

41. Thomas, S. L.: Listening mothers: Oral language development in first grade. Instructor, 77:20-21 (Oct), 1967.

42. Wetzel, R.: Use of behavioral techniques in a case of compulsive stealing. J Consult Psychol, 30:367-375 (No. 5), 1966.

43. Whitney, L. R., and Barnard, K. E.: Implications of operant learning theory for nursing care of the retarded child. Ment Retard, 4:26-29 (No. 3), 1966.

44. Wolf, M., Risley, T., and Mees, H.: Application of operant conditioning procedures to the behavior problems of an autistic child. Behav Res Ther, 1:305-312, 1964.

Chapter Four

THE ART OF BEING A FAILURE
AS A CONSULTANT

QUENTIN RAE-GRANT

CONSULTANTS in mental health have never had it so good. The demand for their services has grown exponentially over the last several years. It used to be necessary in the fifties to conduct a long series of negotiations, and to engage in considerable planning, prodding, and promoting even to get one's foot in the door in such agencies as schools, pediatric hospitals, social agencies, and community services. For survival today, one has to beat off the demands that are coming fast and furious from every direction. The work of Caplan (1961, 1963, 1966) in designating roles that a consultant can plan, the work of pioneers such as the Wellesley Group (Klein and Lindemann, 1961), or the St. Louis Group (Rae-Grant and Stringer, 1964) in the area of school consultation, and the many endeavors in the fifties (Group for the Advancement of Psychiatry, 1956) demonstrated significantly the value of the consultant. The word got around that he had a contribution to make. This position was reinforced by the introduction of agency evaluation mechanisms that gave extra points to agencies who could show that they had ongoing consultation in psychology, psychiatry, or social work — an evaluation that increased their status, and, even more importantly, their ability to command additional funds. The other main influence that has drastically altered the picture has been, in fact, the community mental health movement with its recognition of, and emphasis upon, consultation as a needed mechanism for collaboration with the community to ensure that a community network of services becomes available and works effectively together for the overall mental health needs of an area.

We have heard of the population boom. We are now dealing with a consultation boom; but a boom can always be followed by a bust. There are indications even now that unless we are careful, the backlash from inadequate and poorly conducted consultation may in fact produce just this. Although the title originally suggested for this paper was "Common Errors in Consultation," the present title derives from an excellent and graphic article by Haley entitled "The Art of Being a Failure as a Therapist." Haley, in considering psychotherapy, pointed out how the dice are loaded in favor of the therapist (Haley, 1969). As many of the same factors seem to apply to consultation, the liberty was taken of borrowing and amending the title. This will facilitate discussion of the issue from the viewpoint that while it is difficult for the consultant to fail, strategies are available that can and often unwittingly are used to make this event possible.

With the demand for consultation and with the rather uncritical manner in which it is either being sought or being provided, things are all in favor of the consultant. He brings an "expertise" which agencies have been brainwashed to accept as an essential component for their own operation. He brings the status of an established profession and the immense weight of concern about mental health and its ramifications that is reflected as a general societal value at the moment. There are too few consultants available to go around and the requests that are made are not infrequently of the following nature: "We have this program. We are excited about it. We think it is going to go far to meet the needs but we desperately need from you somebody who can consult with us about the psychiatric, psychological, or social work aspects. Do you know of anybody who could possibly be induced to work with us?"

One notes from this that there is no specification of the qualifications nor little delineation of the expectations, and there is an almost pathetic recognition that consultees may have to be content with whomever they can get rather than being able to tailor their choice to their own needs. The consultant goes in, then, with everything in his favor and really has to work assiduously and studiously to fail. In addition, most agencies, when they are relying on collaboration and help, lean over backwards to be polite, pleasant, and noncritical. The process of evaluation of consultation is poorly worked out, and highly subjective. Therefore, provided the consultant is not outrageously obnoxious or unpleasant, the rating of his work is likely to be favorable even though this may mean considerable distortion of the realities of what transpires in this interaction. How, then, can the consultant-to-be, if he were to attempt to prove that consultation can fail, go about developing a concerted strategy towards this end?

The first essential in the art of failing as a consultant is that of knowing all. The would-be consultant must state to himself, from the beginning, that he knows the answers and that his answers are the only appropriate ones. Thus, he should espouse with conscious deliberation a method of approach that relies solely upon his specific skills and deployment of these skills as the answer to any and all questions. Having decided that his are the answers, he should agree with himself that any and all other answers are to be rigorously and devastatingly dealt with. He should agree that he will use his professional status to enforce his point of view and at the same time to undercut any other alternatives, particularly where these are in conflict with his own preconceptions.

The second way to ensure consultative failure is to know nothing about the consultee; on being contacted by the agency, it is thus important that the consultant decline to find out about the functions, purposes, strategies, opportunities, and limitations under which the agency is functioning. To do so would induce in him perhaps a greater understanding of the problems and resources and a sympathy for the conditions under which the people in the agencies are operating, and would weaken his dogmatic reliance on his authority as an expert. It would also include him as part of the agency and give him his share of responsibility for its operation — a course which would require him to modify, to change and to fashion what he did in order to be consistent with the needs of his "client." This is very similar to the process in individual therapy in which it is stated, often with reason, that therapy will not be embarked upon until those receiving the therapy are willing to accept the preconceptions, the formulae, and the proposed solutions given by the therapist as a prerequisite for any intervention. The consultant should, along this same vein, refuse to define the mandate under which he operates and simultaneously have a covert agenda of his own.

A third most successful maneuver, guaranteed to ensure failure, is for the consultant to seize on the consultation as an opportunity to work out, crusader fashion, some of the very personal feelings that he brings to the situation. As an example, to fail as a school consultant, it is useful not to see the children or the school staff as the people to be helped, but to see the school system as something inefficient, archaic, authoritarian — something to be conclusively modified if not to be destroyed. The problems that the consultant himself had in his school years can now be successfully acquitted through an onslaught on the school system and a working out of old grievances. Statement of the purpose, however, would alert people to this latent agenda. It thus has to be a one-man conspiracy, conspiratorially arrived at and implemented. While it is preferable that the ineffective consultant not even be aware of his own motives, he must avoid at all costs being confronted with them by those who contract for his services or those who are supporting his services or by himself. The consultant must know the answers, attempt to impose them on the consultee agency, and ignore the consultee's ideas, desires, and mandates. Accordingly, he must refuse to permit himself to be educated by the agency. He must stick with his answers, not modify his position, and have the answers ready to the questions before they are raised. Compromise on this is fatal because compromise derives from sympathetic understanding and leads to success.

In defending this position, he must utilize all the skills that he has learned in individual therapy for the management of any potential rebellion in the ranks. To be a failure, the consultant must always be in the right. Just as failure of a case to progress is usually the responsibility of the patient, occasionally of the therapist, but never of the theory, so a consultation that fails to progress is primarily the responsibility of the consultee, rarely of the consultant (unless he is in the training status), and never of the theory and preconceptions behind his mode of operation. A consultant must know the answers to any and every problem. These answers he derives personally and then he imposes them. If these "preordained" answers are not accepted, this rejection must be examined in terms of the resistance of the consultee because of personal hang-ups which are then related to the consultee's failure to follow the valuable advice being offered by the consultant. The responsibility for the consultation and for its success or failure must be placed firmly on the consultee, and the guilt aroused by failure appropriately and lavishly dispensed on his shoulders. The consultant can always fall back on the lack of training of the consultees in the specific discipline of the consultant. He can infer, for example, that a child is failing to progress because he really should have therapy two, three, or four times a week, often of an analytic nature, and that anything less than this tampers with the little individual's psyche. With this mechanism, it does not take long to reduce the consultee to a feeling of inadequacy in what he does, and of agreement with the tremendous dangers of anything other than the magic talisman that the consultant alone can provide. Of course, it is essential in this line of approach that the consultant decline to be involved at all in the demonstration through personal example of the value and methods of such services. It is important that the consultant not recognize that in any consultation there will arrive a point of testing and trial-by-ordeal in which he will be asked to perform on a specific case himself those things which he is preaching to others. He must, if he is steadfast in his desire to fail, refuse to recognize this, or if he recognizes it, decline to accept it as part of the process of developing a constructive relationship.

In order to fail, the consultant must be definite, dogmatic, and unyielding. He must be aware of his status at all times. He must insist on the transposition of methods appropriate in one area (for example, individual therapy) into this other area into which he moves his operation. He can then rally to his aid all the multiple devices of the therapist — the contemplative silence, the provocative nonresponse, the refusal to answer, the penetrating stare, the repetition of the last word or sentence. He then has a number of further choices. If he wishes to be a failure, he should never fail to interpret the consultee's motives — conscious or preferably unconscious. He can fall back on jargon and the use of technical terms with which his consultee is often in no position to argue. He can cover his own confusion about what is going on in the situation by this mechanism, for jargon is a substitute for clarity of thought. If one cannot say something clearly and in plain English, it is more than likely that the person who is saying it has little understanding of what he is propounding. On the other hand, in the first session our failing consultant can launch into a dazzling series of dynamic formulations straight out of Freud and his lesser disciples; this may be very accurate in theory, but of little present relevance and of no meaning in the situation to which he is supposed to be providing aid. He can move further to the subtle and not so subtle suggestion that what the consultee needs is a course of therapy. He does not then deal with what Caplan (1961, 1966) calls theme interference. He translates this into an area with which he is more comfortable; namely, personal dynamics. He can muddy the water between therapy and consultation and confuse each by this concerted cross-purpose approach. He can, and usually will, propose certain lines of action; however, he must guard against these being brought up by the consultee as they are likely to be successfully implemented. He can take those solutions proposed by the consultee and gently, or not so gently, indicate their inappropriateness, naivety, superficiality, or lack of dynamic relevance. He can, in other words, stake out a position of virtue for his solutions and place the consultee immediately on the defensive, requiring him to justify his position against the solid rock of conviction which the expert is expected to provide. Rather than putting his own contribution into perspective, he can assiduously polish his halo and pontificate ex cathedra.

If these methods do not fully succeed, our unsuccessful consultant still has other devices in his armamentarium. He can sulk if his advice is not taken or is not carried through, by refusing to recognize that his role should be to suggest, to aid in the implementation, to be willing continually to review and change, and to work with the consultee on increasingly appropriate avenues of approach.

He can use the ambiguity that is endemic in much of our field to his advantage in either of two ways. He can keep his own statements continually ambiguous with various alternatives that could be maneuvered to mean the same thing; by manipulating the verbal and conceptual symbols, he can make sure that he is never at a loss to show that what was done was not really his advice, or, if the consultee succeeded in spite of his advice, this really was the implication of the consultant's proposed direction all along. On the other hand, he can use ambiguity as something that is inherently to be avoided. He can refuse to help his consultee see that living with ambiguity and working with approximate answers is really the most important process in consultation, and that the continuing involvement in questions by both consultant and consultee is in fact of the essence. Having learned himself, hopefully, to live with and to be comfortable with ambiguity, he can refuse to pass on this lesson to his consultee and can conceal his own feeling of uncertainty with many of the situations that are presented. He can, in other words, present consultation as a static, concrete, and definitive process instead of one in which the dynamic interaction between consultee and consultant is the crux of the creative art of being a consultant.

In order that he be able to continue with this self-defeating task, he must eschew at all points any feedback mechanism for himself. He must make sure that he never honestly reviews in a frank and open manner with the agency just what has transpired and how useful it has proved. He must avoid the development of warm and trusting personal relationships, as this would invite such confidences and exchanges. He must avoid any situation in which he would be required to present a review of what is occurring to colleagues from his parent organization; this might result in playback and perhaps a critical analysis from those who are better equipped to deal with his pseudoprofessional shenanigans. He must insist on "flying solo" before he has learned where the controls and the instruments are. He must also avoid giving a playback of his impressions and ideas to the agency. Confronted with such a demand (and it occurs frequently), the arrogant consultant should immediately turn it into a session for the examination of why such questions are raised and how they derive from individual or agency problems and issues. He must welcome the antagonism that occurs when people interested in having their operation reviewed ask for a frank appraisal and are rebuffed. To give answers at this point means to expose himself and therefore to threaten his position. It means putting himself on the line instead of always having the other person's pathology questioned and examined. This is a remarkably successful device for ending a consultation on a sour note — to turn a legitimate request for evaluation into a session of further nit-picking and consultee examination.

Three final avenues are available to aid in this mission of making a consultation fail: The consultant can accept the all-too-frequent and flattering invitation to get himself involved in the administration of the agency and to propund with authority on areas beyond his competence. He can conspire to cause change when this is neither invited, sanctioned or accepted as one of his tasks. He can form alliances with subgroups within an organization and have great fun wheeling and dealing within agency politics. This ensures that he will take on many of the feelings of agency members about each other and will not be able to deal with these in a constructive and growth-promoting fashion. He can then crown his miserable endeavors by selecting one or two individuals from within the staff for personal therapy. This finally and deftly obscures the essential division between consultation on the one hand and therapy on the other. If he has carried through all these procedures, tactics, and strategies, he may then be asked by the shrewder agency heads to take his expertise elsewhere; however, with the need for consultation as great as it is, there is no guarantee this will happen.

What has been outlined is the great difficulty of failing as a consultant even though many steps and devices are in fact available. The tragedy today is that what has been presented here in a semifacetious way and what everyone may agree should never happen, is in fact happening all too frequently and all too widely, knowingly or unknowingly, in this field of consultation. We are now recognizing that just as therapists are not born but trained, so consultants have to be trained in this particular method of approach. In our training programs we have been, and still are, notably reluctant to provide experience in consultation and to supervise that experience with the same intensity that we give to individual, group, or family therapy. Still firmly held as a belief is the rank assertion that when a man or a woman is competent as an individual therapist he is axiomatically competent in all other areas. The facts simply do not bear out this assertion as has been pointed out by Coleman (1953) and Langsley and Harris (1960). The fact is that training programs have been the last to move in the direction of including training in consultation as a necessary part of preparation for the fully equipped practitioner. They have failed to recognize that just as talking and reading about therapy does not equip a person to be a therapist, so lectures about consultation have little relevance until the person has actually experienced in practice and in vivo those issues alluded to in didactic presentation. We agree that the therapist in training must become involved with patients, make his errors, and learn from his errors. We have not applied, in most cases, the same principle to consultation. Further, with the assumption that the individual trained in therapy is competent in all areas, we have not set up a continuing education and review of consultation methods in our operating agencies. It is essential that the training in consultation be a continuous process with the support for the consultant from a group and the self-monitoring that this method provides (Rogawski, 1968). What we have done is to make people knowledgeable about consultation, rather than to teach them to be consultants.

To remedy this situation we must help people to distinguish clearly between the processes and implications of therapy and consultation. We must help the consultant define his role before he enters an agency, spell out the negotiating process with the agency, clarify his expectations and the agency's expectations and their congruence and incongruence. We have to aid the consultant in working out with the consultee a helping alliance similar to that which we discuss in negotiating a contract with the individual patient or the family. We have to help the consultant recognize that he does not and cannot be expected to have the answers to every question. We have to help him be able to say he does not know, but not to withdraw defensively in the face of this alarming discovery. With regard to training programs, it is essential that these provide their trainees with a proper perspective of what we do not know as well as what we do know, and simultaneously to foster a feeling that continuing involvement and willingness to work with others towards the solution of problems is in itself a major helping contribution. We have to prepare the young consultant particularly, to adopt a position of modesty even at the end of a long, expensive, and arduous training; to help him see consultation as a learning process for himself and a fascinating opportunity to expand, in a post-postgraduate program, his knowledge of fields allied to but distinct from his own professional discipline. We have to induce in him a respect for, rather than a fear of, the contribution of the consultee. We have to help him open his eyes to the skills that teachers, clergymen, and agency personnel have, and the contributions that they often make without having had the advantage of extensive mental health training. We have to induce in the consultant an appreciation of their difficulties and a respect for these as he attempts to work alongside them, and we have to aid and support him in continuing to work with others as together they struggle to deal with the many problems that exist.

For the agency, the other side of this partnership, it is crucial that the contribution asked from the consultant become more appropriate and realistic. He is *not* the answer man; he certainly is not God. He should not be encouraged or cajoled to be either. While he can keep jumping off the pedestal, it is less tiring for all if he is not hoisted up into this position. It is eye level, healthy and at times skeptical and questioning use that makes consultation worthwhile. The opposite — slavish, adoring, bemused or dazzled dependence is as stultifying for the consultee as it is alarming to the consultant. To find the casual comment tossed off in an idle moment appearing next week as agency policy brings forth laughter and tears and probably deserves both.

If the above review seems somewhat harsh in its description of consultation and at times seems to have over-represented its errors, it is only because of concern that we do not fritter away the opportunity that is now being presented to us. This opportunity is to promote a mental health delivery system by which the limited number of personnel in mental health can make their skills available to and synchronous with a much wider helping group. It represents the only mechanism by which we will ever manage to match the needs of the population on one hand, with the limited resources of professional manpower and "know-how" on the other. The invitation is open to us — in fact the demand is pressing — but the consultant is the guest in the host agency and should comport himself with the restrictions, constrictions, and politeness implied by this role. In responding to this demand, we have the opportunity to help ourselves and those with whom we are concerned; we have a responsibility to proceed to do this with the same high professional concern, standards, cautions, and controls that we use in our practices. Consultation is an art, but there is an increasing underpinning of science in its implementation. It is a challenge. It depends even more than individual therapy on the qualities that the individual brings: on his very humanness and ability to work with imperfections of his own and those of his consultees towards the goal of responsibility and shared endeavor in the helping field.

We have been offered the challenge, accorded the invitation and given ample entry. It is up to us, individually and collectively, to ensure that we do not abuse the situation and lose the opportunities that are being presented. The next few years are crucial to the question of whether mental health will continue to have relevance to wide issues and wide groups or whether it will be forced, and by its own mistakes and errors, into an increasingly esoteric and isolated function in our society. The answer will largely depend on the success of our efforts to develop sophisticated and insightful consultation and consultants.

REFERENCES

1. Caplan, G.: Prevention of Mental Disorders in Children, Initial Explorations. New York, Basic Books, 1961.
2. Caplan, G.: Types of mental health consultation. Am J Orthopsychiatry, 33:470-481 (April), 1963.
3. Caplan, G.: Principles of Preventive Psychiatry. New York, Basic Books, 1966.
4. Coleman, J. V.: The contribution of the psychiatrist to the social worker and to the client. Ment Hyg, 37:249-258 (April), 1953.
5. Group for the Advancement of Psychiatry: The Consultant Psychiatrist in a Family Service Agency, GAP Report 34, March, 1956.
6. Haley, J.: The art of being a failure as a therapist. Am J Orthopsychiatry, 39:691-695 (July), 1969.
7. Klein, D. C., and Lindemann, E.: Preventive intervention in individual

and family crisis situations. In Caplan, G. (Ed.): Prevention of Mental Disorders in Children. New York, Basic Books, 1961.

8. Langsley, D. C., and Harris, M. R.: Community mental health activities of psychiatrists. Psychiatr Q (Suppl), 34:314-325, 1960.

9. Rae-Grant, Q., and Stringer, L.: Design for a new orthopsychiatric discipline. Am J Orthopsychiatry, 34:722-729 (July), 1964.

10. Rogawski, A. S.: Teaching consultation techniques in a community agency. In Mendel, W. M. and Solomon, P. (Eds.): The Psychiatric Consultation. New York, Grune, 1968.

SECTION III
The Consultee's View

INTRODUCTION

DISCUSSIONS of consultation usually are organized from the point of view of the consultant. It is he who tends to be concerned with the dynamics of the consultation process and who is interested in measuring the effectivness of consultation. His goals are likely to be considered more important or more fundamental than the goals of the consultee. Training programs are usually directed at developing skillful mental health consultants, and planning is focused on how best to train and deploy mental health consultants.

Yet, the consultee in many ways is as important or more important than the consultant. Without a consultee, there can be no consultation, and unless the consultee properly fills his role, even the best consultant is hampered or made ineffective. The consultee is very often a professional and there is no reason why a standard part of professional training should not be on how to be a consultee. Effective consulteeship undoubtedly requires a number of skills including the ability to abstract and describe the essential elements of a problem, the ability to choose cases which can best be benefited by consultation, the ability to choose among the many bits of advice given by a consultant, and the ability to carry out the consultant's advice.

Each consultee enters the consultation relationship with a set of expectations as well as a professional role, professional background and history of experience with consultation. The consultant must take these into account in determining what advice to give and how to deal with his consultee. What may be good advice and proper support for one consultee is likely to be inadequate or even disturbing for another. Because of the traditional positions of consultant and consultee with respect to each other, it is not easy for the consultant to be aware of inadequacies in his own performance or dissatisfaction with him on the part of the consultee. It is with this in mind that the following chapters have been written. The consultant needs to hear what the consultee's view of him is and to consider what changes in his own role are necessary so that he may better meet the consultee's needs.

The consultee group is truly a varied one. While consultants come from a small number of mental health professions, consultees can vary all the way from an individual with a Ph.D. or M.D. to an individual who has not graduated from high school. Consultees may be policemen, bartenders, teachers, nurses, halfway house administrators, volunteers, and even secretaries and receptionists. This range of interests, training, and levels of responsibility presents a particularly difficult problem for the consultant.

In the following chapters, two diverse examples of consulteeship are presented. In the first, Beard, a social worker and director of Fountain House, describes his experiences. Fountain House is primarily a club of ex-psychiatric patients with a daytime and weekend program. The program is mainly social and vocational with some apartments available for those who do not live independently. Fountain House was founded by an ex-patients' group seeking to band together in a nonclinical setting but in such a way as to provide mutual support. In some of its elements, Fountain House appears to be anticlinical in that members are deliberately not treated as patients, and manifestations which in another setting might be considered as illness are dealt with socially. Yet even in Fountain House there is a need for the advice of mental health professionals. These professionals will always have a role in Fountain House albeit a limited one. Beard describes the reactions of his staff and his members to the psychiatric consultants which Fountain House employs.

A completely different setting is described by Robinson and Falconer. Robinson, a child psychiatrist, and Falconer, a teacher, have worked together in a consultation program in the suburban school system of Clarence, New York. Although Robinson has been the consultant, he writes here from the point of view of the schoolteacher and attempts to describe some of the pressures on the teacher. It is clear that much of this pressure comes from acceptance of a professional role and an internalization of professional values, many of which are based on conditions of a previous era or upon idealization of the teaching situation. Under such circumstances, one important role for the consultant is to help the teacher examine some of these beliefs which may be inappropriate or disruptive to effective functioning.

Chapter Five

MENTAL HEALTH CONSULTATION
TO SCHOOLTEACHERS

JAMES A. ROBINSON and JUDITH FALCONER

AS the responsibilities of the schools in our society increase, it is the teachers who bear much of the increased burden in the form of longer hours, more advanced professional training requirements, relatively decreased facilities and financial support, and increased emotional pressure.

Attempts have been made to help teachers with this burden. Professional teacher preparation, curricula and in-service training programs provide teachers with increased technical skills. Teaching machines and other devices free teachers to perform an ever-widening range of tasks.

However, as a consultant to public schools and as an elementary schoolteacher, respectively, we have been impressed by the fact that teachers are usually offered little systematic assistance in dealing with the increased emotional stresses which accompany these new responsibilities. In the absence of such assistance, it is important that teachers nevertheless learn to cope with these problems.

Most teachers overcome external problems created by the educational environment. They acquire the skill necessary to circumvent unreasonable or impractical administrative regulations. Some teachers transfer when they find it difficult to work in a particular school. Others remain in the same school, assuming that the difficulties which they encounter are due to their personal and professional shortcomings but, nevertheless, reaching some accommodation with the system. All teachers occasionally feel they are doing an inadequate job.

Clarence, New York, is a small town at the outskirts of the

suburbs of Buffalo, New York. The school system consists of 4500 students and 250 teachers distributed among four elementary, one primary, one junior high, and one high school.

Ten years ago the school system social worker requested private consultations with one of us (Robinson) while he was in full-time private practice. We had formal contacts for seven years. The school system wanted more.

Eighteen months ago, it became possible to offer eighteen three-hour sessions, one session every other week. Time and money were agreed upon and a series of single session consultations began. Attendance at each session included the social worker, school psychologist, and between ten and twenty teachers who were requested to come by the principal. The principal also usually attended. Each meeting was devoted to discussion of a problem pupil. This consisted of fifteen minutes of summaries of the history and psychological test results, twenty minutes of anecdotal reports (what the child did, what the teacher did, and what either helped or made a situation worse) by teachers who knew the child, and then a one and one-half hour discussion. Following the meeting, the school social worker and I had a postmortem. Later in the evolution of the relationship, we had brief sessions before the group meeting in which she described the teachers in advance.

What were the details of the hour and a half discussion? At various times, chosen on the basis of the affective response and interest of the teachers, different stereotypes of behavior were examined. The "lazy" child could be seen as a compulsive child fearful of making a mistake; similarly, the "procrastinator." "Attention-seeking," "aggressive," "works only in a one-to-one relationship," and "hyperactive" evoked clarification of the manifestations of limit-seeking, separation-anxiety, organic and constitutional or environmental contributions to bothersome classroom behavior. Teacher affect was gently identified: anger, resentment, sadness, affection, and sympathy. Tentative explanations, where seemingly appropriate, were offered. The frustration of teacher failure, fear of loss of control of angry impulses, fear of firmness, and especially the effects of teacher fatigue were introduced as a basis for teacher feeling and reactions. Constitutional factors such as varying activity levels in children, the effects of physical size differences, and physical attractiveness were considered. The possible influences of family styles and a possible correlation between the teachers' knowledge of the parents and the child were included in the clarification of reasons for behavior.

Seldom were there decisions about courses of action. Occasionally, a decision could be made about the need to refer a child and his family for treatment to a clinic. The emphasis, however, was on what the teacher herself could do to deal with the immediate problem. Because of clinic waiting lists, a referral to a clinic was tantamount to washing one's hands of the problem. This was explicitly stated.

Following each session, an evaluation sheet loaded in the direction of criticism and suggestions was given to each teacher to be answered anonymously. Later, each teacher was asked if the consultations in which she had participated were helpful in understanding and handling (1) the particular child discussed, (2) any other child with whom there had been a problem in her class but who had not been discussed, and (3) problems in the teacher's personal life.

These are the responses of the forty-four teachers attending from one to three sessions. Five expressed great satisfaction, four were extremely dissatisfied and the rest felt the sessions were either very helpful or slightly helpful. (On the basis of the generally favorable acceptance of the consultation, the program has been increased to thirty sessions for this academic year.)

Most informative are the comments which I shall list, first the reasons for the favorable response, then the reasons for the negative response and finally, the teacher criticisms generally.

I. Favorable

A. Specific suggestions helpful (twice).

B. Makes me reevaluate my reactions and be more patient (twice).

C. Helpful to know family background (six times).

D. Experts don't know all, I feel more adequate about myself.

E. Liked use of everyday language.

F. I am not afraid to be firmer.

G. Any and all information helps.

H. Helped me personally (four times).

II. Unfavorable

A. Should see and treat the child.

B. Want more individual contact with the consultant.

C. Resented interpretations without seeing the child; therefore, interpretations had no validity.

III. Criticisms

A. Want more concrete suggestions (four times).

B. Meetings shouldn't be on class time.

C. Need to know student's background at beginning of the year (five times).

D. Smaller group would be better.

E. Wish for in-service training.

F. Should see child personally before consultation.

G. What is this — sensitivity training?

H. Need coffee and cake if after school.

I. We should cover only one child, not two

J. Sessions too long.

Summarizing these comments, the repeaters were (1) request for specific answers; (2) acknowledgement of usefulness of background information; (3) helped me personally; and (4) helped me to be more patient or firmer.

Some general impressions are described below. The teachers of kindergarten through fifth grade for whom we have provided consultation are more receptive, responsive, and open in their consideration of emotional factors affecting school performance. These teachers seem to be less threatened and more sympathetic to the child with problems in the classroom. Since their pupils have not yet begun to have different teachers for different subjects, the teachers are able to know well their thirty to thirty-five students. The teachers of children in the higher grades become increasingly content and academic success-oriented and the teacher's frustration level rises to the extent that there is less interest in understanding the significance of emotional factors. By high school, the lines of battle seem drawn and more teacher feeling arises from the threat of loss of control which is expressed as an authoritarian and punitive orientation to teaching. Middle and high school teachers also have contact with up to one hundred fifty different children and hardly get to know each child.

Much of the stress on teachers arises from several common but irrational assumptions under which they operate. We feel it is important to identify these assumptions, to show their effects upon teachers and students, and to demonstrate their irrationality. We hope the resulting self-awareness will provide teachers with better understanding of their difficulties and increase both their professional effectiveness and personal satisfaction. These irrational assumptions are listed below.

1. THE TEACHER WHO IS COMPETENT AND WORKING TO CAPACITY CAN DO THE JOB WITHOUT HELP. Teachers are now provided with specialists in many fields: the reading teacher, school psychologist, school social worker, physical educator, music and art teachers, and the curriculum consultant are some examples. They exist, not because the teacher is incompetent, but because no single teacher is capable of developing expertise in all areas of education. Many teachers mistakenly assume that to utilize these resources is to admit incompetence. The converse is true: the teacher who coordinates the resources of a variety of specialists is much more competent than the loner.

2. A GOOD TEACHER SHOULD BE ABLE TO WORK WITH ANY AND EVERY CHILD. If students were assigned to a particular teacher on the basis of rational criteria, this might be true. In schools where the unique capabilities of each teacher are taken into account in scheduling classes, teachers are more effective and satisfied; this is seldom the method used. Personality development takes place to a large extent as a result of the individual's environment and experiences. In some cases the environment and experiences of particular students and teachers will be so different that their goals are too divergent for cooperative behavior to occur. Teachers must be willing to admit that they cannot be all things to all students. Conflicts will arise; situations will develop where a teacher cannot work effectively with a particular student. This does not reflect on the competence of the teacher. In many cases it is possible to "work with every student" only if the student's creativity and personality are stifled.

3. THE TEACHER MUST BE FRIENDLY AT ALL TIMES. Teachers who exercise sufficient emotional restraint in the

classroom to suppress all personal anger, depression, frustration and fear, may also limit their expression of affection, satisfaction and the fact that they care about each student. Students should find learning an exciting challenge, not a task. The emotionally sterile classroom denies this challenge. Teachers are not paragons of virtue; they are human beings. If human contact were not an important part of child development, our public schools could be turned over to the teaching machine, which often is more effective in teaching factual material. A significant teacher function is to help children learn how to work with others. The teacher can and should provide the role model and a classroom environment in which this important interpersonal learning can occur.

4. "THE TEACHER NEXT YEAR WILL BLAME ME IF THE STUDENT HAS NOT LEARNED ALL HE IS SUPPOSED TO KNOW." Although many teachers cynically deny that they believe this argument, they unconsciously seem to accept it. Students learn at different rates and at different times. Grade school students take reading readiness tests so the proper time to introduce this skill can be determined. In most other curricular areas, we ignore the readiness of the student and accept the blame for failure to learn. This is obviously irrational.

5. MANY TEACHERS ASSUME THAT IF THEY FAIL IN A PARTICULAR AREA, THEY WILL BE REVEALED AS THE FAILURES THEY ALWAYS FEARED THEY WERE. If teachers operate on this assumption, whether on a conscious or unconscious level, the effect on students can be damaging. The teacher who is able to admit failure in a certain area, on a certain day, or with a particular student can convey to students that failure on one exam, in one course or in one grade is not an irrevocable catastrophe. Students must be taught to challenge failure, to understand why it happened and to defend against its recurrence in constructive ways. Teachers who cannot bear their own failures cannot provide good role models for their students.

These are some of the irrational and often unconscious assumptions upon which teachers operate. Many teachers also have attitudes which make their jobs more difficult. It is important to state some of these attitudes and to bring them out in the open for inspection.

Teachers' assumptions about the result of failure often provoke an attitude of guilt. Our society evaluates the teachers' effectiveness by their students' grades and test performance. Those who produce students who receive the most academic honors and awards are considered the most competent teachers. Since most students never reach the top of the class, success really lies in developing the ability of each student. The motto of the State University of New York, "Let each become all he is capable of being," should be the goal of each teacher.

A second attitude which makes teaching difficult is the teacher's identification with a particular child. Most teachers find a few children in each class particularly attractive or unattractive. Upon introspection, they usually find that these children remind them of something or someone in their past; the emotion tied to that person or event is transferred to the child. Teachers often find it difficult to discipline children they like and to reward children they dislike when such identification exists. Disliked students initially try to gain the teacher's favor but eventually give up and behave in accordance with the teacher's attitude. Favored students often become behavior problems when they learn that the rules do not apply to them. If teachers are aware that this identification takes place, they will be more able to control its negative effects on students and themselves.

Teachers are often unaware that they tend to displace their personal problems onto students and the teaching environment. Teachers often find the student who insists on having his own way particularly frustrating. Is this because the student can oppose the rules of the classroom, but the teacher cannot oppose the policies of the administration? On a more mundane level, the teachers who had flat tires on the way to school, or who have "volunteered" to chaperone the next school dance, often express their suppressed anger and hostility towards the students. In a more positive vein, the students have been known to comment, "It must be payday, the teachers are almost human today." Teachers cannot leave their personal problems on the doorstep of the classroom. They must, however, be on guard against using students to resolve these problems.

A final example is the tendency to stereotype students.

Teachers encounter many cliches about students and youth: "There is no such thing as a bad child; no kid really wants to learn; kids from that neighborhood are always difficult to teach." The danger of such stereotypes is that they evoke automatic responses. Teachers must remember that each student is an individual and entitled to be treated as such.

We have stated some of the irrational assumptions and dysfunctional attitudes which make teaching more difficult. What can teachers do about them?

In the first place, teachers must explore the assumptions upon which they operate. Unless they can identify irrational assumptions, they can do little to make their jobs less difficult.

Secondly, teachers must explore their attitudes toward themselves and their roles as teachers. How many of the above attitudes do they hold? What can they do about them?

Finally, the teacher is left with the question, "Whom can I ask for help?" Although students are an obvious source, they are often overlooked. Teachers assume that students are unaware of classroom and school problems; yet anyone who has talked with students realizes that they are aware that these problems affect the learning process. Students across the country are asking for an opportunity to improve their schools, communities and nation. Teachers who listen when students talk about education will learn a great deal which can help make teaching less difficult.

Teachers often benefit from the advice of their colleagues as much as from the advice of a trained psychiatrist in consultation sessions. Teachers are the experts in dealing with education problems; interpersonal techniques, psychological knowledge and a somewhat more detached view of the problems can be provided in consultations. It is the teachers, however, who must decide what problems exist, explore methods of dealing with them, and eventually solve them. Far too often, the "go it alone" assumption prevents working together to solve mutual problems.

Teachers can make their jobs less difficult. Some of the ideas presented here provide a starting point. Students, teachers and administrators, working together in an atmosphere of respect, cooperation and trust, can vastly improve our educational system.

Chapter Six

PSYCHIATRIC CONSULTATION FROM THE CONSULTEE'S POINT OF VIEW

JOHN BEARD

IN describing the experiences we have had for the past fifteen years at Fountain House with psychiatric consultation, I think it would be helpful to first review the Fountain House setting and its programs of psychiatric rehabilitation.

Our agency was established in 1948 as a nonprofit, voluntary organization for the express purpose of facilitating the community adjustment of psychiatric patients following their release from public and private mental institutions. We are located in New York City, just a few blocks from Times Square. In 1966, we completed the construction of our new clubhouse — a six story, Georgian Colonial building designed to accommodate over four hundred men and women at any one time. Some three hundred patients, known as members, are active in our day program, and another six hundred men and women attend our evening social and recreational programs. Social workers, psychologists and rehabilitation counselors largely make up our staff of sixty full and part-time workers, but increasingly we utilize nonprofessional mental health workers, many of whom are former members of Fountain House. Our 1970 budget of approximately $800,000 makes possible our rehabilitation programs and our education and research activities.

Almost 90 per cent of our members have a diagnosis of schizophrenia. Most have undergone multiple or long-term hospitalizations and almost all, at intake, are financially dependent upon family or public welfare. The majority become active members soon after leaving the hospital, but we encourage membership for those still hospitalized who can come to the agency during the day, returning to the hospital at night. Close to one hundred referrals are made each month from mental health facilities serving New York City.

Since 1955, our clubhouse has been open seven days a week. Social and recreational activities, such as dancing, discussion groups, dramatics, photography and bridge, are available in the evenings and on weekends. The evening program is believed helpful to members when they first obtain full-time employment and cannot attend during the daytime hours. Membership at Fountain House is continual in that a member can return to the setting at any time. Frequently, one comes back just to visit. Others reappear at a time of personal crisis, such as when a job is lost or when there is a reemergence of illness.

The daytime hours at Fountain House are used for the purpose of developing the work capacity of the individual, so that gainful employment can be secured. Members do many things at Fountain House during the day. We have not had to be creative in finding things to do. Each day we prepare the food we eat, keep our house clean, and take responsibility for the many clerical activities which need to be performed. In our view, most of our members at intake have established a pattern of accommodation to disability. Yet there are many things a member can still do which are in keeping with his interests, strengths and capacity and which, when performed, can legitimate his participation.

Our members greet visitors and new applicants, for example, and take them on tours of the facility. They handle our busy switchboard, maintain attendance records, and make home visits to members who have become isolated from Fountain House. With two hundred and fifty lunches to serve each day, our members must plan menus, purchase the food at the local A & P store, prepare the food in the kitchen, provide table service to everyone, and do the necessary cleaning up each day after lunch. They operate a snack bar on the top floor of Fountain House, which is open mornings, afternoons and evenings. They perform all kinds of maintenance tasks in the building and we work together keeping it clean. They go to the post office for the mail, type letters, run the mimeograph machine and perform other clerical tasks. They publish a daily newspaper, engage in tutoring, assist in our research work, and are extremely active in developing audiovisual materials for our training and education programs. They help explain to visitors what we do, give talks in the community, and appear on radio and television.

Members run our beauty shop, the library, our music room; they operate a thrift shop on Ninth Avenue, just around the corner from Fountain House. In all these activities, members and staff work side by side, be it in the kitchen or in the thrift shop.

We try to develop our relationships to each other through our joint participation in all of these activities. Visitors to Fountain House see firsthand what we are trying to do. They see a lot of people being very active and they hear arguments, words of appreciation, praise and satisfaction. They also see disappointments and frustrations, rewards and pleasures.

In the course of developing our day program, we found that many members, in a few months or a year, were able to move on to jobs of their own in the community. Others, however, made an excellent work adjustment at Fountain House but were unable to separate themselves from our environment and assume independent employment. To help overcome this difficulty, we initiated in 1957 a program which we call "transitional employment." We believed that private enterprise was an untapped resource in the rehabilitation of the vocationally disabled and that a program could be created whereby private enterprise could serve as a bridge or ramp from Fountain House to regular employment in the community.

Today, one hundred and fifty Fountain House members in our day program are spending part of their day working in some forty business and commercial firms in New York city. Each of these employers has reserved one or more of their jobs for the use of Fountain House. Wages range from $1.85 to $2.35 an hour. An eight-hour day serves two members — one in the mornings and one in the afternoons. Typically, our members remain on the job for three or four months. The job is then available to another Fountain House member who is usually introduced to the job by the member who has successfully completed it. Over a period of a year, our members earn close to $300,000.

A member may work as a messenger or file clerk, a typist or a keypunch operator. Some do factory work or assembly work;

others, porter work. All the jobs are simple and do not require special skills. We have selected such jobs on purpose. While the work may be beneath the educational skill of the member, essential features of the work situation are present: money, fellow employees, a boss, the requirement to be productive and to meet work standards. In all of our placements, a staff worker first performs the job to acquire a direct experience of what the member must do if he is to be successful.

Some of our members cannot handle a placement and must return to Fountain House. Others may go through two, three or even four placements. Approximately one half are able to move on to full-time jobs of their own from transitional employment. As you would expect, it is not easy for our people to give up readily a pattern of financial dependence and vocational disability.

While most members are on placement work on individual jobs, about one fourth go to work each day from Fountain House to what we call "group placements." We have four such group placements — one in a large department store, two in cafeteria or restaurant settings, another in a distribution center of a national merchandising company. In these group placements, from six to ten members work together on the job as a group. We are solely responsible for the selection of members, often filling in employment forms right at Fountain House. One of our group placements can be easily visited. It is a Chock Full O'Nuts store on Seventh Avenue, between 28th and 29th Streets. With the exception of two employees, all the workers are members of Fountain House.

It was necessary for us to develop group placements for those members who seemed to need the security of performing productive work in the presence of other Fountain House members. They did well in their work at Fountain House, and we saw no reason why a similar work environment could not be established in industry. While on-the-job supervision is provided by regular employees in two of the firms, an innovation in supervision has occurred in two of the placements. At Sears, Roebuck and Co., the supervisor is a regular employee who was a former Fountain House member and who had achieved her vocational adjustment through the transitional employment program. At the group placement at Chock Full O'Nuts, the manager of the store is a full-time member of our staff, having been employed by Fountain House because of his extensive experience in restaurant management. We receive reimbursement, by the way, for the management function he performs.

Another service of Fountain House concerns the living accommodations of our members. As an alternative to the traditional halfway house, we have rented some twenty-five apartments in various neighborhoods of New York City which we then make available to patients leaving the hospital who have no home to return to, or to those members in the community whose housing is inadequate. Typically, two members live in an apartment and share responsibility for its care. By pooling their financial resources they have the advantage of a kitchen, living room, bedroom and bath. We have been able to secure from the community most of the furnishings of the apartments through our thrift shop. About 85 per cent of the rental cost is paid by the residents. Our charitable dollar, therefore, goes a long way with respect to securing better housing for our members.

Withing the last two years, we have intensified our efforts with respect to education and research. A small brownstone immediately adjoining our new clubhouse has been secured and our members are active participants in our research work, as well as our growing educational programs.

Our experience with consultation goes back to 1955 at which time our agency, for the first time, had the services of a psychiatrist for four hours a week. From our founding in 1948 through 1955, there was a resistance to having psychiatrists, regardless of function, active within the setting. It was believed that the environment should be as free as possible from any suggestions of clinical services. The founding effort was to set up a new environment, one which would bear little resemblance to the mental health services which Fountain House members had experienced in the past. Initially, the effort was made to run the program exclusively with members and volunteers. When it was concluded that at least minimal staff were needed, the decision was made to employ staff who had had little or no experience in working with the mentally ill.

By 1955, it was decided that members by themselves were

unable to operate and maintain a rehabilitation program, and that not only was a staff needed, but one which had experience in working with the emotionally ill. Furthermore, the agency rejected the view that a social-recreational club was sufficient, in itself, to enable the socially and vocationally disabled mental patient to achieve a successful community adjustment. With an operating budget of $37,000 a year, an entirely new staff was secured including a psychiatric consultant. New programs were initiated. As the programs and the staff expanded, a second psychiatric consultant joined Fountain House in 1963, a third in 1968.

Clearly, we have had an experience with psychiatric consultants, and for the past couple of months we have been trying to clarify this experience for discussion. A starting point for us was to go to our staff, and to our members, and ask them for their views and observations concerning the role and function of our three consultants. Our survey was done with some thirty staff members and just under one hundred Fountain House members. We tape-recorded their comments but did not have intensive or in-depth interviews. Many responses were secured. To begin with, staff and members made a number of comments which revealed their lack of awareness as to what our three consultants do at Fountain House. We collected such phrases as the following:

> I have never had any contact with them . . . I am not sure what they do . . . I haven't been here long enough to know anything about them . . . I don't think I've ever talked to them in my life . . . I really have no idea what they do . . . I've never referred any members to them . . . I've never used them . . . I've never seen them . . . I've never had any contact with them . . . I don't know what the key thing is they do here. . . .

On the other hand, the helpfulness of our consultants was described in rather simple, direct ways.

> They help me . . . They help us . . . They help with medication . . . They help with emergencies . . . with referrals . . . and they help when you don't have knowledge . . . They help our students . . . our members who don't have doctors . . . our staff when they get disturbed or confused . . . They help the volunteers . . . help get patients out of the hospital . . . help to get them in . . . and help decide if we can handle someone at Fountain House. . . .

They help write papers . . . help sustain us . . . help us prepare
organizational charts . . . help when legal problems come up . . . and
help keep records . . . They help balance the program . . . Yes, I think
she is a very helpful person . . . They are most helpful when we are at
a complete loss. . . .

We also found that the word "give" came up in many of the
responses. The consultants were described over and over again in
terms like the following:

They give prescriptions . . . give pills . . . give on-the-spot help . . . give
treatment . . . give advice . . . give us some good ideas . . . give a
professional balance to our work . . . and give their signatures on all
kinds of forms. . . .

Consistant with the feeling that our consultants "give" in their
work at Fountain House, there were many positive feelings
expressed, such as follow below:

They are warm people . . . I feel he is a friend . . . They make you feel
more secure . . . I get a lot out of them . . . It's nice to have them
around. . . .

A number of our staff and members emphasized that our
consultants were really not a part of our setting and the distance
from Fountain House was perhaps a good thing.

I wouldn't like it if they were here all the time . . . It's good they're
not permanent or full-time . . . I'm glad they have a practice on the
outside . . . They are not intimately involved in what we do here . . .
You are able to use them because they are not a part of Fountain
House . . . It would be like a hospital if they were here all the
time . . . I think they're helpful, but at a distance. . . .

Our survey elicited numerous views of ambivalence towards our
consultants, often viewing the presence of the psychiatrist as
symbolic of the reality that many patients will inevitably fail in
their post-hospital adjustment.

I guess I like them being here . . . I don't object to having them
here . . . It is like a last resort when you have to see them . . . You
only see them when you are in trouble . . . You only see them when
you cannot be handled. . . .

Most of the staff and members of Fountain House viewed
psychiatric consultation in terms of "their personal relationship"
to the consultant.

They are responsive to our questions . . . They let us use them as a

> sounding board ... show interest in what we are doing ... and don't treat us like three-year-olds ... I think we reinforce each other's views ... I think we get biased once in awhile and they help correct this ... It is not like when we had a nurse here and everyone wanted to lay down all the time ... It is good to have someone to talk to ... I think most of us wish they were here more often. ...

Rather detailed description was also secured as to the variety of functions which our consultants performed.

> They teach us ... attend our staff meetings ... answer all kinds of questions about symptoms and drugs ... bring in experts to talk to us ... prepare written evaluations ... get information for us from hospitals ... tell others what we do here ... check out new employees ... sign all kinds of letters to the Department of Welfare, aftercare clinics and other agencies ... They are the best able to get information from doctors. ...

But members and staff were not without suggestions as to the specific changes which should occur in what the consultant does at Fountain House.

> They ought to spend part of their time doing what we do ... They ought to serve lunch once in awhile ... They ought to talk more with social workers than with the members ... They ought to see more of the members who pace around all the time ... They ought to spend more time talking with us, the members, rather than staff ... The trouble is they don't have enough time to talk. ...

Regardless of the views expressed, we believe that the comments of members and our staff recognized the complex role which the consultant performs in our agency.

> I think they make us legitimate in the community ... They know how to treat Fountain House as a social agency, not a medical service ... They are willing to handle emergencies ... We go to them when no one else is left ... Sometimes they substitute for one's own psychiatrist ... Their main job is to help the social workers help us ... You can always get their reactions to our ideas, and our proposals, and not feel put down. ...

These then were the varied comments of our members and staff concerning psychiatric consultation at Fountain House. In the discussion remaining, I would like to phrase a series of questions which, in the view of our supervisory staff, are relevant to fundamental aspects of consultation and which if answered in the affirmative, express our orientation to the consultation process.

With increasing numbers of psychiatric patients leaving hospitals and returning to the community, is there a need to develop more effective services which will facilitate the community adjustment of such patients? Are agencies such as Fountain House important resources in a national effort to provide more effective services? Will the staff of such facilities tend to consist of a variety of personnel, ranging from trained social workers and psychologists to mental health workers, including individuals who may have been emotionally ill and who have important contributions to make? Will patient services in such settings be inevitably provided by such staff? Can the efforts of such mental health personnel, through innovation, evaluation and research, create the needed body of knowledge which is presently lacking? Can consultation with others — be it medical, psychiatric, architectural, financial or other such inputs — be productive in the practice of the individuals responsible for the day-to-day delivery of services?

As to psychiatric consultation, can it become a threat to the leadership of the agency and to its staff? Is it relatively easy for consultation to create dependency and a lack of staff responsibility for the delivery of services? Can the expertise of the consultant, or a mental health worker, be greater than the skill of the individual staff worker and is there a risk that such expertise can foster staff dependency, and even accumulate a caseload for the consultant?

Conversely, might the ideas of the consultant at times prove to be less creative, relevant and effective than those of the consultee? Are not the qualities sought for in staff similar in many ways to what is hoped for in the consultant — maturity, self-awareness and perceptiveness?

Is it clear that the consultant is not the supervisor, the executive, or the staff worker? If the consultant assumes a management role, does this not threaten and weaken the agency's leadership? Is it essential that the consultant not be responsible for a worker's performance? Is the consulting relationship essentially one where the knowledge and experiences of two individuals interact so that one of the individuals may initiate a plan of action which will help lead to a solution of a problem? Should not large emphasis be placed on the importance of a collaborative effort?

Can differences of views be expressed? Can it be done in a temperate manner and can it emphasize the advantage to agency personnel in having the benefit of opinion without the requirement that it be followed? Must differences of views and of opinion constitute a challenge to the authenticity of the worker's alternatives? Must consultation automatically eliminate the legitimacy of other alternatives? Is there a temptation to follow the imagined preferences of the consultant?

Will the consultant interact with staff who vary widely as to professional skills? Will such interaction be adjusted so as to facilitate the better functioning of the less to the most skilled worker? Can the consulting relationship exist even though the consultee has far greater skill in his work than the consultant might have were he a worker in the setting? Should the focus in consultation be in terms of what the worker is capable of doing, rather than what might be done ideally? If consultation is viewed as a growth process, does this mean in retrospect that a consultant will do certain things in the initial phases of his work which he will not do at a later time? Does the level of consultation reflect the degree of learning and experience which has occurred on the part of staff and supervisory personnel?

Must the model of consultation be sufficiently flexible with respect to time, availability and problems, needs and crises? Does one model of consultation apply to all settings? Should the utilization of consultants be primarily a reflection of the increasing presence of consultants in mental health facilities during the past decade, and the availability of funds for such services? May not consultants have special areas of consulting interest — research, education, program development, administrative procedures? Lastly, is not the satisfaction of the consultant related to the growth which might occur with the consultee through the consultation process?

As indicated, we would answer all of these questions in the affirmative. I would not, however, suggest that no additional discussion is required. Since the founding of Fountain House in 1948, psychiatry has had a significant influence in our growth and development. Since 1955, psychiatric consultation has been a permanent and growing function in our staffing pattern. It has never lessened our sense of responsibility nor reduced our satisfactions in what has been accomplished. I think it is probable that we are unable to spell out clearly the ways in which the consultation process has enhanced the functioning of our agency but I believe that this is as it should be, for it is not the object of consultation to have the consultee understand and identify the contribution which the consultation process may be providing to the agency and its programs, to its staff, and its clients.

SECTION IV
Consultation and Its Relatives

INTRODUCTION

T HOUGH mental health agencies vary greatly in structure, purpose, size and staffing, they all tend to include certain fundamental activities which deal with influencing behavior. Foremost among these is psychotherapy — "an effort directed at discovering, understanding and changing intrapsychic dynamics" — as Taintor puts it in the next paper. A second important activity certainly is supervision — the administrative process involved in seeing that the work of the agency is properly done; and the professional or disciplinary process involved in seeing that therapist-patient/client relationships follow theoretical precepts.

Although superficially psychotherapy and supervision seem to be quite distinct, particularly in psychodynamically oriented agencies, they have much in common. As activities they are both attempts to control behavior. The theories underlying them may be similar or the same.

A third important fundamental activity is education and training. Most agencies carry on some sort of in-service training for their staffs, no matter how highly professionalized the staff already is. Many agencies also offer public mental health education. This activity may include lectures, brochures, brief courses and more recently, sensitivity type groups. This general area of activity is of a different nature in terms of design and underlying theory than the others under discussion and so it will not be dealt with further.

Finally, the fourth fundamental activity is mental health consultation. This is the newcomer to the group. Often included with education (as, for example, in the federal regulations for support of community mental health centers) it is not yet as widespread as the others. But consultation is spreading. It can safely be predicted that before much longer, most mental health agencies will be providing consultation for their communities.

Consultation, like psychotherapy and supervision, is at first glance a distinct activity. On more careful examination, it too has much in common with the others. Consultation, psychotherapy, and supervision are the mental health triplets.

Yet, on still more careful consideration, it becomes clear that emphasis on the similarities and neglect of the differences is a dangerous practice.

As Taintor points out, professionals highly trained in psychotherapy easily fall into a pattern of dealing with and understanding every relationship as a therapeutic transaction. However, therapy supposes a particular relationship between the participants and requires a considerable amount of room for the patient to maneuver outside the therapist's knowledge or control. Such conditions are not present in supervision or consultation. Dealing with a supervisee or consultee as if he were a patient at best leads to ineffective work. At worst it can lead to the end of the relationship and perhaps a punch in the nose for the therapist-would-be-consultant or therapist-would-be-supervisor.

In discussion of relationships among professionals, one further point, commonly neglected, needs to be mentioned. Professionals, by virtue of being professional, are required to be loyal to ethics, traditions and precepts which go beyond the regulations of any agency or orders of any supervisor. Psychiatrists particularly, as physicians, are trained to take personal responsibility for the decisions made in regard to a patient. The orders of a supervisor or the regulations of an agency do not relieve the physician of this responsibility. Consequently, the physician must have the last word regarding his patient. Neither the physician nor the patient can be considered cogs in a machine or raw materials in the bureaucratic process.

By extension as well as by independent tradition, the other mental health professions have similar prerogatives, although to a lesser degree. Any discussion of the functioning of mental health personnel must take this anomaly into account. Professionals who are employees cannot act like other employees and simply take orders. They have the right and the responsibility to exercise professional judgement regardless of whether it is in conflict with orders or policies.

In Chapter Seven, Dr. Zebulon Taintor systematically analyzes the differences among psychotherapy, supervision, and mental health consultation. Taintor, a psychiatrist with experience both as a community mental health service administrator and a director of a psychiatric residency, knows well the area which he discusses. He devotes particular attention to "the contract." This increasingly popular term is used to describe the usually unwritten agreement between agencies or professionals. Like the unwritten constitution of England, it is a figurative document whose intricacies and details may go beyond that of a written statement.

In Chapter Eight, Gertrude Flynn, an experienced psychiatric nurse and teacher of psychiatric nurses, presents a unique description of the area also covered by Taintor. Her paper is shorter and more allegorical than most and so it requires intensive study. The reader will be well repaid for the effort required to understand and contemplate the implications of this paper.

Chapter Seven

PSYCHOTHERAPY
VS. SUPERVISION
VS. CONSULTATION

ZEBULON TAINTOR

CONTRASTING psychotherapy, supervision, and consultation provides an opportunity to define by distinction. "Psychotherapy" is used in this paper to denote an effort directed at discovering, understanding and changing intrapsychic dynamics and patterns. "Counseling" denotes specific recommendations for action and behavior without a conscious confrontation of intrapsychic variables. Of course, good counseling takes intrapsychic variables into account and psychotherapy hopefully leads to different behavior. The choice of one rather than the other involves a determination of a client's needs and potentials. A choice of psychotherapy assumes the prime importance of intrapsychic variables and the patient's ability to understand and change; a choice of counseling may assume a need for action to remedy a specific situation or the patient's inability to change or understand intrapsychic variables. "Supervision" is used here to encompass two rather different activities: (1) the usual range of administrative necessities involved in getting work done within an organization, and (2) case supervision in psychotherapy, casework, and so forth. "Consultation" is used here in relation to our specific subject, mental health consultation. Traditionally, consultation in psychiatry had to do with a face-to-face confrontation with a medical or surgical patient. The field of medical consultation is broad and possesses its own copious literature. The purpose is to evaluate a patient diagnostically and offer specific suggestions for treatment. Schwab (1968) has written a helpful handbook covering traditional psychiatric consultaton.

Here we shall deal with mental health consultation which involves "indirect service," hearing about and helping the consultee to deal with the case rather than having a direct confrontation with the person identified as a patient or client. Often the distinctions among these types of activities are confused, and a blurring of heuristic boundaries leads to mishandled and disastrous operations, administrative upheavals, and dissatisfied consumers of service. Some of the problems have to do with the development of supervisors and consultants from professionals who were first psychotherapists. People believing in psychotherapy, i.e. the primacy of intrapsychic variables, are likely to extend its concepts and practices into other areas. A psychotherapeutic approach may become part of a person's style in dealing with many situations in life. In psychiatry the belief in the primacy of intrapsychic variables stems from the revolution brought about by Freud's genius. Most mental health professionals accept at least some Freudian insights, and the existence of an unconscious is unquestioned and increasingly documented by dream investigators and others. Although psychoanalysis has lost some of its luster as a universally applicable treatment modality, its concepts are ever more broadly applied. The interpretation of unconscious needs and determinants of behavior is widespread, and is probably second only to the giving of simple advice. Interpreting behavior rather than directly attempting to control it is probably seen by most mental health professionals as both more democratic and sophisticated. Psychodynamic interpretation is thus invested with more charisma, and the ability to interpret behavior can become an important part of a person's identity. The interpreter is nonauthoritarian, since he does not tell people how to be, yet he is in a superior position because of his apparent awareness of unseen and powerful forces. Training in psychotherapy, especially in psychoanalysis, can be seen as providing a human cosmology in that why people are the way they are is explained logically and persuasively. The convinced psychotherapist sees the amount of psychopathology in the population as accountable for the agonies of the human condition, and sees attacking that psychopathology as his unique duty. However, the obvious importance of intrapsychic variables in determining behavior should not be the sole criterion for attack, because mutability may be low. For example, educators aware that drug dependency blocks educational progress have embarked upon therapeutic enterprises that further confuse the schools' socializing and educative functions to the detriment of the latter.

Another factor relating to the impact of training in psychotherapy has to do with an awareness of the influence of personality factors on the work of a mental health professional. Psychotherapy involves the exploration of "gut" feelings and involves a belief that strong personal feelings must be engaged for a transaction between people to be really important. Thus, a supervisor or consultant may be geared to elicit those feelings.

In consultation, Caplan counsels against this, recommending "professional armour" (1970). The consultant or supervisor who disregards Caplan's advice finds himself confronted with difficult questions of confidentiality and administrative and work priorities versus personal priorities. What is he to do with personal secrets he has been told that have direct bearing on his role as a supervisor or consultant? Sometimes, personal information is offered by the consultee as a manipulation. This information then cannot be utilized either psychotherapeutically or in the consultation and thus limits the options of the recipient. For example, suppose someone whose job performance is inadequate tells a convincing hard-luck story to his supervisor. The supervisor must balance the achievement to be gained by getting the job done against that to be gained by being compassionate and helpful. Suppose a worker says he cannot work well because of his intense and apparently psychodynamically well-founded dislike of a co-worker whose job performance is excellent?

A situation not infrequently encountered in consultation is that of an inadequate therapist striving for self-respect and competence. The consultant, aware of the therapist's shortcomings, may be sufficiently impressed by potentials that could be achieved easily if only certain intrapsychic blocks were removed. If he confronts these directly, he is embarking upon psychotherapy. If he decides to approach tangentially by getting more information, he may be told in strictest confidence that the therapist and patient have an after-hours social relationship that is alleviating (or enhancing) the therapist's problems as well as the patient's. Distinctions between social and therapeutic relationships have become blurred with the introduction of befrienders, therapeutic communities (Rapoport and Rapoport, 1959), and sociotherapy. Such personal communications must be handled somehow and give rise to transference and countertransference feelings and problems. How does a therapist feel later if he is encouraged to communicate but is subsequently rejected? How does the consultant feel if he finds out that the therapist and patient are skiing together? Sleeping together? Taking drugs together? Solicitation of these feelings is all too easy for a consultant who is also an accomplished therapist. Such an individual who is eager to help or who may feel uniquely qualified to be of great help, increases these problems dramatically.

These problems can easily arise when consultation is confused with supervision. Consultation that turns into supervision can duplicate or undercut the agency's administrative system, resulting in double messages and divided loyalties if the consultant is charismatic. If he insists on acting as a supervisor without the implicit consent of the consultee, he will be resented and the consultation will fail.

Brockbank (1968) describes a consultation that was unsuccessful for a related reason — the supervisor's absence engendered discussion of him. Garrett (1956) has suggested that tendencies to encourage administrative acting out can be minimized by having the consultee's supervisor present during consultation. While time-consuming and probably likely to mute communication between consultee and consultant, this suggestion emphasizes the fact that consultation is at least a triadic relationship. Individual psychotherapy is, of course, dyadic, and it could be argued that supervision is largely so. Other members of what is at least a triad in consultation are the consultee's client, the consultee's supervisor, and other members of the agency structure.

Because of the complexities of his relationship, the consultant may find himself hamstrung by people he never sees. He may be regarded as a hatchet man for the agency administration or may find himself chairing gripe sessions directed at the administration, even though he cannot handle the complaints. Because of the paucity of cues in consultation, he may be unaware that the information be receives is determined by alliances within the agency. Political issues that arise may extend far beyond the agency. These have been described by Papanek (1968).

Because of these confusions, Rapoport (1970) has found it useful to contrast the three activities we are considering here as to goals, purpose, contract, and nature of the relationship, as well as to content and focus of communication. I shall add several other variables, some of which owe their existence to historical precedents. These are summarized in Table 7-I.

PURPOSE

The purpose of dynamically oriented psychotherapy is to help a person confront directly his feelings and his defenses against his feelings. His symptoms and defenses are delineated and coping mechanisms are developed. Specific psychotherapy goals are set eventually and both the client and the psychotherapist can state what insights have been achieved and what feelings have been explored.

Supervision is not meant to involve such feelings. Its purpose is to provide guidance and surveillance. Professional skills are developed and the job is seen to have been done.

The goals and purposes of consultation are less easily described. Overtly, the consultee is to be helped with a work problem, usually by clarifying its nature, underlying assumptions, and possible solutions. Covertly, however, the consultant may be involved with trying to deal with underlying problems or attitudes that unconsciously interfere with usual work performance.

CONTRACT

A contract is the agreement that governs the activity involved. There are agreements about activity time, place, payment, and authority.

Explicitness

Contracts involve expectations; unspoken expectations often

TABLE 7-I

COMPARISON OF PSYCHOTHERAPY, SUPERVISION, AND CONSULTATION

Parameter	Psychotherapy	Supervision	Consultation
Purpose	Direct confrontation of feelings; examination of intrapsychic	No direct confrontation of feelings; instead, get the work done	Help with a work problem; covertly to ease anxiety and promote competence
Contract a) Explicitness	Negotiated explicitly as part of the process	Explicit as part of the supervisee's job	Only partially explicit; covert purpose not verbalized
b) Payment	From client; therapist dependent on client	From agency; long-term, not dependent on supervisee	From agency; short-term, dependent somewhat on consultee
c) Time	Varies, brief to long-term; set by client	Long-term; not set by supervisee	Varies; set by agency with consultee; exposure to any one case usually brief
d) Authority	Derived from client; equal or superior, but unenforceable	Derived from agency structure; superior and enforceable	Equal; any superior status given by consultee
e) Nature of relationship	Complicated, well-studied process	Specific, goal-directed	Often vague, complicated process that is beginning to be studied
f) Content and focus of communication	Broad; may be bizarre and irrational	Goal-directed and rational	Overtly goal-directed, but covertly looking for a hidden process
Institutional and disciplinary relationships	Excluded from a dyadic relationship	Usually clear; supervisor and supervisee usually of same discipline	To be worked out; disciplines usually dissimilar, institutional relationships, informal coalitions, political issues
Number of people reached	Few	More	Many, but possibly in too dilute a fashion
Evaluation	Subject of considerable study; being refined	Defined by specific agency practice	Difficult; apparently doomed to inexactitude

are the seeds of future problems. Contracts should be negotiated explicitly in all three areas, but consultation is almost routinely expected to do more than what is specifically agreed.

The contract in psychotherapy becomes increasingly explicit. Initially, the psychotherapist may find himself dealing with suspicious biases and magical thoughts that must be worked through as part of therapy. A patient may be expecting to fall in love with the psychiatrist. An apparently sophisticated client may later reveal a profound belief that psychotherapy will not work for him. The patient knows he is to discuss all thoughts, feelings, ideas, and actions that seem bothersome or relevant. He is to build understanding in order to make better choices.

In supervision, the contract involves the supervisee working within the framework of choices acceptable to his supervisor. Personal feelings may not be irrelevant, but they are not always explored and often must be suppressed.

In consultation, the contract has to do allegedly with a brief or relatively infrequent structured encounter with a specific problem. As other possible agendas are sensed by those involved, renegotiation and specification of the contract may become desirable.

Payment

Usually a patient pays his psychotherapist according to an agreed upon hourly fee schedule. The agency provides salary or wages to the supervisor irrespective of his supervisee, while an agency's financial arrangement with its consultant can be quite variable – by the hour, by the job, by the year. Payment determines authority and leads to a dependency by the psychotherapist and consultant on their clients. In a clinic, psychotherapist and counselor are sometimes not dependent on clients for payment. Sometimes this leads to an obvious lack of concern for satisfying patients, but the operation still depends on the patient's voluntary return for more service and has few sanctions to apply in the event of nonappearance. The consultant is dependent on the agency for renewal of a contract that is usually of a shorter term than that of the supervisor. The supervisor is the most independent of the three and usually possesses such authority and ability to invoke sanctions that the supervisee is dependent on him.

Time

Some psychotherapy can be very brief and even combined with consultation (Karp, 1966), but most courses of psychotherapy are longer. Supervision is usually long-term. Consultations can feature one hearing of a particular case while others can be longer, but they relate to an agency rather than a specific individual. In psychotherapy, the client eventually determines specific appointments and how much more time he wants while an agency does the same for its consultant. The supervisor determines himself when and how long he will meet with his supervisees.

Authority

Both psychotherapy and consultation feature nonauthoritarian relationships between helper and helped. The consultant cannot tell his consultees what to do; the relationship is one of help proffered, but no acceptance is required — a situation similar to psychotherapy. Supervisors, on the other hand, are shackled with the responsibility of making sure things are done. This may lead to some people preferring to be supervisors rather than consultants, although not necessarily because they are authoritarian personalities.

The psychotherapist and the consultant are usually nondirective and may even pride themselves on being nonthreatening, while the supervisor is the boss of the supervisee. Thus the responsibility for use of the helping person rests with patient and consultee, but not with the supervisee. It is the supervisor's role to make sure that he is properly utilized.

Nature of the Relationship

In psychotherapy, the patient attributes considerable expertness and authority to the therapist, and transference and countertransference phenomena are expected. Three phases ensue: acquaintance, combat, and alliance. In supervision, the supervisee is not expected to reveal his inner feelings toward his supervisor. Workers do not have to know each other personally or understand each other. Authority is not just attributed by the supervisee, it is tangible and derived from the organization. Authority is exercised in evaluation, review, and direction. Positive relationships hopefully will abound, but will be based on respect rather than love. Consultation is defined as a nonauthoritarian relationship. The consultant is chosen from a group outside the authority of the agency and is often of a different professional discipline from the consultee. The relationship is more equal, or at least low-keyed despite an attributed authority of expertness. Of course, the good supervisor is aware of the interplay of his and the supervisee's personalities, but we accept the truism that one does not have to like someone to work for him. In consultation, more emphasis should be placed on identification and counteridentification with consultee and agency. These have been well discussed by Simons (1965).

Content and Focus of Communication

In psychotherapy, though the patients' communications may be bizarre and irrational, they are at least highly subjective and laden with feelings. Devices such as free association, hypnosis, and psychodrama are directed to reveal what is hidden from the patient himself. In supervision, communication is expected to be goal-directed and rational. Personality is relevant as it affects work performance, but is usually handled in pragmatic terms. In consultation, communication may vary according to the style of the consultant, but is usually goal-directed with a receptivity for clues of a hidden process. We expect consultants to get at what is not discussed openly.

The breadth of the client's problems discussed varies considerably. In psychotherapy it is generally broad. In supervision, it can include all of the supervisee's professional activities for which the supervisor is responsible. In consultation, the range is narrowest. Consultation is usually sought on a particular case that is chosen because it is not run-of-the-mill but rather is an exception. The consultee may then offer only a segment of that case to be discussed, thus further narrowing the range. Sometimes expectations go beyond the purpose of the consultation surface (Hitchcock and Mooney, 1969). Of course, the person being supervised has clients and so does the consultee. However, information about these other clients is filtered through the supervisee and consultee on its way to the supervisor and consultant. The filtering process usually involves opinions, and emphasis is determined in part by the supervisee's or consultee's feelings and approaches to his client. A literature is developing about consultee types and dynamics that resembles descriptions of patients. Mumford (1968) has described three commonly encountered types of schoolteachers and the sorts of issues they present in school consultation, while Papanek (1968) has discussed consultee types generally found in consultation. In supervision, a frank discussion of the supervisee's feelings may be important to his handling of the agency's client, and a discussion can be brought about through the intervention of the supervisor. In consultation, Caplan (1970) has suggested that the consultee's feelings can be somehow dealt with without being openly discussed. He suggests that this procedure avoids embarrassment and prevents the relationship from becoming psychotherapy. He suggests ways of avoiding psychotherapy, pointing out the lack of safeguards, contractual ambiguities, and so forth. We see the alleviation of anxiety as a significant function of the consultant as well as the therapist. Some sort of answer must be given to direct questions. Just as one swallow does not make a summer, a discussion of a person's feelings does not make ongoing psychotherapy inevitable.

INSTITUTIONAL AND DISCIPLINARY RELATIONSHIPS

The institutional relationship is not important between psychotherapist and client and is understood between supervisor and supervisee; namely, both are attached to the same institution and the supervisor has authority over the supervisee for the tasks with which they deal. The consultant must define his institutional relationship. Similarly, the patient is rarely of the same discipline as his therapist while the supervisor and the supervisee usually share the same discipline. In facilities staffed by multidisciplinary treatment teams, there may be a difference in disciplines, but this is usually attenuated by a general blurring of disciplinary roles. In consultation, however, consultant and consultee do not usually share the same discipline. Differing areas of competence usually facilitate asking for help if there is mutual respect for each other's talents, but can lead to problems of status, personality, and professional affiliation (Boehme, 1956).

Agency structure, informal coalitions and political issues may determine the sort of patient treated by an agency and perhaps the mode of treatment offered, but are basically of little significance in the dyadic relationship of psychotherapy. Similarly, supervision generally resolves these problems by defining procedures that handle the issues even while not necessarily confronting them.

NUMBER OF PEOPLE REACHED

The number of people reached has been of increasing concern in a time of manpower shortages and the drive to increase services to all people. Psychotherapy admittedly reaches a small group of people. Supervision offers a senior mental health professional a chance to transmit his talents, intelligence, experience, and professional stance to those in supervision. They fan out and reach more clients than the senior man could possibly have encountered by himself. In consultation, potentially even more people are contacted because consultants are utilized by nonmental health agencies such as the police and the schools that have dealings with many more people. This also offers the prospect that mental health problems can be recognized and dealt with early. In this respect, the argument for consultation is most impressive. There seems to be a chance to improve every aspect of society and to reestablish communication among balkanized groups. On the other hand, dilution and overextension can engender a sense of meaninglessness.

EVALUATION

Evaluation is a central problem in consultation. Outcome in psychotherapy is a much-studied problem. Evaluation of supervision is usually specified in a detailed fashion by the supervisor's agency. Evaluation of consultation, however, poses several problems. The process is new, and techniques must be developed. Relationships are informal and not authoritarian, so a failure of accomplishment may be hard to localize. Exposures are often brief and therefore hard to get at. Finally, consultation sets out with a hidden agenda that cannot be evaluated directly because it is not openly discussed. Favorable reports from consultees may not tell the whole story. A consultant's ability to develop the hidden agenda may be successful but lead to overall failure – a successful operation, but a dead patient. Brockbank's (1968) experience is probably just one of many examples. More often, consultation may be an apparent success while perpetuating agency drift and self-satisfaction, a pleasant conspiracy of apparently dealing with the issues. The maturation of the field of mental health consultation depends upon the development of effective evaluative techniques. Only then can the mental health consultant be certain his work will survive and go beyond being regarded as a fad.

CONCLUSION

The differences discussed are shown in Table 7-I. Consultation is, of course, unique, but seems to bear a stronger relationship to psychotherapy than to supervision. We would like to suggest an historical similarity based on our review of the literature. Initially, there was a spate of articles extolling the virtues of consultation and offering guides on methodology. Recently, there have been articles emphasizing the dynamics (Hitchcock and Mooney, 1969; Papanek, 1968; Berlin, 1960). Yet, there has been almost as little word from the consultees as from the patients. And, like psychotherapy, there has been little research into quantifying events beyond the anecdotal level. We hear more about dynamics than about whether or not consultants are doing the job. Some consultants are probably right in saying of an agency, "They had unreasonable expectations," just as some patients are properly called unmotivated, but still, it would be better to see some data dealing with the task in hand.

REFERENCES

1. Berlin, I. R.: The theme in mental health consultation sessions. Am J Orthopsychiatry, 30:827-828, 1960.
2. Boehme, N.: The professional relationship between consultant and consultee. The use of the consultant: workshop. Am J Orthopsychiatry, 26:241-248, 1956.
3. Brockbank, R.: Aspects of mental health consultation. Arch Gen Psychiatry, 18:267-275, 1968.
4. Caplan, G.: The Theory and Practice of Mental Health Consultation. New York, Basic Books, 1970, pp. 24-26, 97-106.
5. Garrett, A.: Psychiatric consultation. The use of the consultant: workshop. Am J Orthopsychiatry, 26:234-240, 1956.
6. Hitchcock, J. and Mooney, W. E.: Mental health consultation. Arch Gen Psychiatry, 21:353-358, 1969.
7. Karp, H. N.: Combined mental health consultation with crisis therapy. Arch Gen Psychiatry, 14:536-543, 1966.
8. Mumford, E.: Teacher response to school mental programs. Am J Psychiatry, 125:75-81, 1968.
9. Papanek, G. O.: Dynamics of community consultation. Arch Gen Psychiatry, 19:189-196, 1968.
10. Rapoport, D., and Rapoport, R.: Permissiveness and treatment in a therapeutic community. Psychiatry, 22:57-64, 1959.
11. Rapoport, L.: Personal communication, 1970.
12. Schwab, J.: Handbook of Psychiatric Consultation. New York, Appleton, 1968.
13. Simons, R.: Mental health consultation and the problem of counter-identification. Compr Psychiatry, 6:410-418, 1965.

Chapter Eight

THE ROMANCE OF CONSULTATION

GERTRUDE E. FLYNN

W E are concerned with attempting to distinguish between supervision, psychotherapy, and consultation. As a person who at different times wears three hats, with each of the hats relating to one of these functions, I would like to share with you how I view them. I will try to point out some of the things which help me to remember which hat I am wearing and how so far I have avoided becoming a "Mad Hatter."

I view psychotherapy as having many of the characteristics of a really good daughter-father relationship. The daughter looks to the father for guidance and love, being appropriately dependent at times, but ultimately an independent individual. She goes through a period in which daddy cannot be wrong and a period in which the "stupid old man" knows nothing. She takes on many of the basic values that the father has, tries them for fit, accepts those that are most complementary or most needed, and rejects those which are just too foreign or quite comfortable. The father is caring but not smothering, concerned but not too directive, flexible but not excessively permissive, vulnerable at all times but with sufficient self-confidence that he survives and at times thrives. The daughter-father relationship is intense but has physical limitations. There is, of course, some authority of the father over the daughter, but its implementation is better carried out by expectations rather than by direct control. The relationship of a caring father and a receptive-responding daughter is also characterized by a mutual respect with well-understood responsibilities for each person. Like psychotherapy, the daughter-father relationship becomes less intense and in a sense terminates and goes on to a different type of a relationship when the daughter goes on to a man of her own. True, the new relationship does not act as a substitute, but rather the new relationship has much of its success due to the warmth of the earlier loving experience.

Supervision, on the other hand, I see as a rather comfortable relationship, having characteristics of a good marriage of ten to twelve years. The man and wife are in harmony with one another, sharing many similar experiences, but always preserving their own identity. They are able, in a sense, to "psych out" one another, but do not neglect to consistently validate their observations and to provide generous "feedback." In this kind of a relationship there is not one dominant partner, but each knows a bit more than the other about different things. There is little competition and, in fact, there is a delight as one partner progresses in competence with the understanding and interest of the other. In a marriage of this type, there is not the emotional dependency we observed in a daughter with her father, but rather two individuals more equal in their contribution to the relationship.

In this ideal marriage, or the supervisory process we are discussing, there is a common sharing of a philosophy or beliefs which with experience, one with another, are somewhat modified while extreme positions are abandoned. There is comparatively little crossing over of fundamental identity groups such as race (in marriage) or discipline (in supervision), but this is becoming a little more frequent in liberal communities. In marriage, the contract is clearly understood at the onset although as in supervision, nonanticipated conflicts may demand behavior more oriented toward crisis intervention or unfortunately, at times, premature termination. In marriage, the behavior is defined, the techniques are clearly understood and the obligations fully accepted if the contract is to be a success. Marriage, like supervision, eventually terminates once the task has been accomplished, with each being a better person for having experienced the other.

The consultation process I perceive as different from psychotherapy which I described in terms of the daughter-father relationship or supervision which I compared to a good marriage. Rather, consultation can be described as a love affair of the French variety. Evidently, an affair with a French lover (and I neither confirm nor deny primary data) is something quite unique for a woman. The lover tells the woman really nothing startling or new about herself, but rather has the woman accept herself in an entirely new dimension. He comes across very strong at first, is extremely stimulating, exciting and provocative. Contact with him makes the situation, or life, seem entirely different, and that which was mundane or perhaps even hopeless, suddenly becomes worthwhile.

The French love affair depends on several factors which are equally important in the consultation process. One, the point of contact – the entry into the system – is vital. Certainly an invitation, even if only a perceptive glance by the woman, is helpful. Secondly, there is a time element that must be considered. Given the right time in the life of the woman – or system – and the spadework for the success of the adventure is already accomplished. Thirdly, there is a certain charisma, an aura that surrounds the relationship. True, it may not be reality oriented, but it should not be destroyed until it has served its purpose, i.e. to arouse interest and encourage trust. Like the love affair, consultation should have a contract that clearly states what is expected of one another, the limitations of the involvement, the shortness of its duration and the understanding that win, lose or draw, there are no regrets. I am told that in a good French love affair the techniques are varied, the influence tremendous and the rewards very gratifying. Perhaps that is what makes the consultation process so very inviting for many of us.

SECTION V
Consultation Training

INTRODUCTION

ALTHOUGH George Bernard Shaw made the oft-quoted comment, "He who can, does. He who cannot, teaches," there is much to be said for the other point of view. In many situations, it is the teacher rather than the practitioner who has the harder task and it is the teacher who faces a realistic evaluation of his work while the practitioner rarely is critically examined.

Consultation is an example of one such situation. In practice, the consultant often faces a group of individuals who are naive in the area of mental health and whose natural inclination is to look upon the consultant as godlike and all-knowing. When standing before such an admiring audience, who rarely, if ever, question or talk back to the consultant and who never report to him his mistakes or inadequate advice, the consultant is inclined to believe that he has indeed taken on some godlike qualities. An essential element of being godlike is not having to account for what one does. Being placed in such a position makes it simple to forget if one is doing nothing or is not really clear on the effectiveness of one's work. Only the students, then, trying to understand what the consultant really does, are likely to probe beneath the consultant's armor and make him aware of his weaknesses.

In the case of consultation, for example, one glaring weakness is in the area of theory. Why does consultation work? How often and with what kinds of persons should it work? With which individuals should it not work? Rare indeed is the consultant who has answers to these questions and who, as he practices his skills, remains aware of the uncertain foundations of his work. Consultees are not likely ever to raise these questions. Students will do so all the time.

The training of mental health consultants is an important issue today because mental health consultation has become an accepted part of community mental health programs. Yet, as in most aspects of community mental health, there are almost no individuals formally trained to do the work. Many of those presently practicing have developed expertise from reading and then trying out their skills in an unsupervised clinical situation. Such a training approach is inefficient and quite possibly ineffective. If consultants are to be trained in numbers large enough to meet the need, some formal training programs must be developed. Some fundamental decisions must be made about how consultants are to be trained. For example, should mental health consultation training be part of every program to train mental health professionals, or should mental health professionals of diverse backgrounds come together for advanced training? What is the best preparation for consultation? Is a clinical background helpful or would a more academic training in behavioral science be best? How much of consultation should be taught in the classroom and how much should be taught as an on-the-job apprenticeship?

In their paper, Babigian and Pederson begin to address some of these problems. Obviously, they do not have all the answers but they have been training consultants for a number of years as part of a residency program in a department of psychiatry. As a multidisciplinary team, they offer their experiences to begin the discussion and to help arrive at some decisions regarding the training of mental health consultants.

Chapter Nine

TRAINING MENTAL HEALTH CONSULTANTS

HAROUTUN M. BABIGIAN and ANDREAS M. PEDERSON

TRAINING programs for mental health consultation must consider the transmission of a conceptual framework and the development of an appropriate training methodology specifically geared to the consultation process. Goals of this training are to prepare mental health professionals to function as consultants in their general field of practice, and hopefully to minimize and prevent problems encountered in consultation programs. Because mental health consultants work in a variety of settings with many different individuals and problems, a general training program for mental health consultation is a very difficult topic to outline in terms of a specific curriculum. Some of this difficulty can be attributed to divergent ideas as to what mental health consultation is and the skills an individual must acquire to perform as an effective consultant. Initially, therefore, we think it would be appropriate to indicate what we feel mental health consultation is in relatively general terms and then proceed to discuss how individuals might best be trained in this field.

Regardless of the specific definitions of mental health consultation, there are several common denominators for discussing this area. First, the consultant might be any mental health specialist: psychiatrist, psychologist, psychiatric social worker, mental health nurse or nonprofessional mental health worker. Second, the consultee potentially could be anyone involved in help-providing community programs. Third, the major orientation of consultation is that of indirect intervention or as Caplan (1963) describes it, "consultee-centered case consultation." Fourth, the emphasis in consultation programs is on prevention rather than on specific treatment. And last, an impetus to mental health consultation is the increased leverage it gives to mental health professionals in a community through the use of other people who are already involved in helping agencies in that community. Consultation can be viewed as a major bridge between the traditional clinical-treatment model and the community-prevention model which has been developing in mental health fields throughout the 1960's. This emphasis represents a major orientation shift which has been receiving increased attention both in mental health literature and in mental health care.

Usually, when one speaks of mental health consultation in community mental health, one is referring to consultation which is focused on expanding mental health care and services through the utilization of individuals not necessarily engaged in mental health programs. Caplan (1965) defines this type of consultation as

> ... a process of interaction between a mental health specialist and a member of another profession in regard to the mental health aspects of the latter's work with a client or program, in which the consultant helps the consultee improve his effectiveness in handling the current problem and at the same time helps him increase his understanding of the issues involved so that he may be able to deal more adequately on his own with similar problems in the future [p. 94].

In the pamphlet "Consultation and Education," prepared by the National Institute of Mental Health (U.S. Department of Health, Education and Welfare, 1967) consultation is defined as

> ... a fairly complex, two-way process in the art of helping people – the systematic use of mental health knowledge to achieve the greatest good for the greatest number ... (mental health consultation) is generally understood to be a voluntary relationship between two or more professionals whose exchange of information, cooperation and collaboration helps solve an existing or potential problem [p. 3]

One can discuss the conceptualization of mental health consultation, its values, benefits, and impact on a community without difficulty, but it is quite a different problem to formulate how one actually trains individuals to become mental health consultants. The type of training program designed for mental health consultation is dependent upon the designer's personal orientation, the availability of experienced training staff, the cooperation of community agencies for field placements, the sophistication of the trainees and the incorporation of such training into existing mental health curricula. Because many questions presented to the consultant require that he call upon his totality of past educational experiences, and as Sarason and Ganzer (1969) point out, because most of the consultant's work is done in an *ad hoc* fashion, the development of any training manual or program of "how to do consultation" becomes very difficult. Even when one develops and implements a training program there may be problems. The *Report of the Boston Conference on the Education of Psychologists for Community Mental Health* (Bennett, 1966) cautions that developing a training program which is too rigid could in itself stifle change and flexibility of approach which is needed if the training is to help the consultant reach the needs of different communities and changing populations. Knowledge of community consultation is still in the developmental stages. It is quite possible that what we feel is important today may have to be discarded tomorrow. Therefore, any training program for mental health consultation must be flexible, able to incorporate new knowledge, and willing to experiment with new and different approaches. This requires that the training faculty be especially open to new learning experiences with the willingness to adapt to change.

Consultation and education is one of the five essential service areas of community mental health centers. The National Institute of Mental Health estimates that at least 10 to 20 per cent of staff time in these centers is devoted to this service area (PHS Publication 1478, 1967). Kern (1969), however, points out that mental health consultation as a chief component of community psychiatry has only recently gained acceptance as a respectable psychiatric activity. He estimates that NIMH is presently supporting at least twenty different residency training programs in community psychiatry, all of which have some consultation training. These programs vary considerably as to the emphasis placed on consultation as opposed to other areas of community psychiatry. For example, the GAP report, *Education for Community Psychiatry* (1967) provides a list of institutions involved in teaching community psychiatry throughout the United States; of the sixteen different institutions listed, only ten outline consultation training per se as a primary objective in their training programs. The rest imply that while consultation training is included in their general community programs, it is not seen as independent or necessarily as more important than any other area of emphasis. Even with the increased emphasis on community psychiatry and psychology and the development of consultation training programs in certain educational institutions, there remains a large proportion of mental health professionals who do not receive consultation training during their mental health education experience. Hassler (1965) conducted a survey which included twenty-two approved psychiatric residency training centers in Massachusetts. Fifty per cent of the residents indicated they were receiving little or no training in consultation theory and techniques, and 90 per cent indicated that training in epidemiology, program evaluation, or public health principles was minimal or nonexistent. However, he also found that 68 per cent of the residents said they were currently interested in community mental health and would probably remain so in their future practice. Within the area of community mental health itself, 67 per cent of the residents were most interested in consultation theory and techniques.

With the increased interest demonstrated by mental health professionals in community programs and the increasing demands for consultation services, there is a definite need for more attention and emphasis directed to training in community mental health including consultation and other closely related areas such as epidemiology, community organization, biostatistics, program evaluation and public health principles. Several imaginative and innovative programs which attempt to provide this type of training are currently operational and have been described in the literature. These programs range from intensive workshops such as those described by Ozarin (1963) to specialized year-long training programs following at least two years of residency training outlined by Kern, Spiro and Kolmer (1966), Kern (1969) and Caplan (1965). Other programs such as those proposed by Daniels and Margolis (1965) and Daniels (1966) stress the need for including consultation training as part of the core curriculum for all psychiatric residents during their first two years.

The preparation of a specific training curriculum is not the only area for consideration when developing a mental health consultation training program. Other factors influence training programs and may determine the success or failure of even a well-conceived and meaningful program. Therefore, the remainder of this paper focuses on some of the issues which must be considered prior to the development of a training program for mental health consultants, as well as a description of the training program at the Department of Psychiatry of the University of Rochester School of Medicine and Dentistry.

Issues to be considered prior to the initiation of training programs for mental health consultations are listed below.

1. THE UNIVERISTY. The university is the primary source for training all mental health professionals, yet the overall emphasis and push for consultation and education programs came from the community mental health movement outside the university, propelled by the Federal Government through the Mental Health Centers Act of 1963. Most university departments were not involved in the conceptualization of this program and resisted in varying degrees any changes in the operation of their traditional training systems. Most university departments considered community mental health centers to be primarily service-oriented and thus not easily amenable to the traditional university approach where education and research have priority over service. In university training programs, services are organized around the educational goals of the institution as contrasted with the philosophy of community mental health centers where education and research have to evolve from and revolve around basic principles of comprehensive service to a defined population. Because of these differences, most university departments that have assumed responsibilities for community mental health centers are currently struggling in search of a compromise to avoid a two-system faculty, one service-oriented and the other training- and research-oriented. Romano (1966) in discussing this issue states:

> ... as a medical school, we know that our usefulness would be seriously impaired and our survival in danger should we become exclusively a community clinical service station. At the other

extreme, if we were to become exclusively a research institute, detached from our environment, we would fail in our principal obligation, that of education [p. 36].

He goes on to emphasize the need to achieve a proper balance between these two extremes. One way of achieving this balance is the inclusion of community training programs as integral parts of the general residency or postgraduate training program. All mental health professionals should be taught the basic principles of consultation and given an opportunity to practice them in a closely supervised setting. More advanced and specialized training may come after this based on the interest of individuals and geared towards the preparation of future teachers and researchers in consultation and community psychiatry. The bulk of consultation is and will continue to be carried out by professionals who are not necessarily consultation specialists.

We feel that it is imperative for the concerned faculty in community mental health programs to work closely with the faculty group that designs the postgraduate curriculum. This helps to assure representation in the planning group and makes it possible to proceed into the development of training programs in community mental health, including training in consultation, as integral parts of the general training program of the institution.

2. TRAINING METHODOLOGY. There is a basic difference from traditional methods in the training of individuals as mental health consultants that warrants close consideration and examination. The traditional training of the clinician in medicine, psychiatry, psychology, social work and nursing is based on the direct supervision of the trainee while providing diagnostic study and treatment to a patient or a group of patients. The trainee provides the basic service to the patient and is supervised closely by a teacher who may also use direct observation to help in the educational process. Such an arrangement is not possible nor advisable in a consultation setting where the goals and contractual agreements between consultant and consultee vary and are different from the clinical setting.

Kaplan (1969) discusses these differences and recommends that schools of medicine follow the model of schools of public health and social work in developing structured relationships between the training school and community agencies which may participate in the training process. Although such an arrangement resolves some of the problems, we do not feel that the supervision of the trainee should rest totally in the hands of an agency or its personnel. The trainee should not identify with an agency or its representatives but with the faculty members from the university who are the consultants to that agency.

The faculty involved in the training of mental health consultants should be actively engaged in the community with ongoing consultation programs, and must assume direct service responsibilities. Therefore, we recommend that the faculty develop ongoing consultation service programs with agencies with the agreement that these programs will be used for the training of professionals. These programs will be totally viable even without the services of trainees. This kind of arrangement is a complete departure from the traditional orientation of the university in which clinical training programs are designed to accommodate available trainees without the faculty necessarily assuming a direct service responsibility.

3. COMMUNITY MENTAL HEALTH CENTERS. Community mental centers, university-based or otherwise, open their doors with consultation and education services as one of the five major sections of their organization. Two problems arise immediately with the inception of a center: (a) Few professionals on the staffs of community mental health centers have been trained in consultee-oriented consultation theory or techniques. Yet most of these centers rapidly attempt to implement "consultation programs" in the communities they serve. Because of the inexperience and lack of preparation of the staff, many of these programs have been designed entirely along the lines of traditional models of patient-oriented consultation services. This has resulted in programs which focus on organized case referral and direct service with which the staffs are most comfortable. Unfortunately, these programs neglect the broader implications of consultation services, particularly consultee-centered consultation. To develop appropriate and effective consultation programs, we feel it is as important to train the staff of community mental health centers in consultation as to develop general consultation training in a

university setting. This will allow the participation of center staffs in the education of mental health professionals through the use of their consultation programs. (b) Consultation programs are frequently developed prior to the education of the community regarding the goals of the center and its available services. Usually, communities are able to grasp the significance and need for the four basic direct services. However, the goals and benefits of consultation and education services are more difficult to understand. For the development of effective consultation programs and training it is imperative that centers educate the community and facilitate community representation and involvement in their operations.

4. THE TRAINEES. While we feel that mental health consultation is an important area, this does not necessarily mean that those being trained hold the same attitudes. To assure the effectiveness of a training program, interest has to be cultivated through the practical demonstration of relevance to trainees. Goldston (1964) has pointed out that residents frequently have the notion that community psychiatry and consultation are practiced by psychiatrists who are far less capable than psychiatrists with large private practices. In many settings, the trainees do not see the principles of community psychiatry as relevant, and have difficulty developing positive attitudes about mental health and preventive measures as contrasted to mental illness and specific treatment modalities. Some of this difficulty results from the manner in which new programs have been introduced into existing training programs. In some cases they have been "tacked on" without proper integration into existing programs and, as Kaplan (1969) points out, staff and supervisors frequently have not been experienced. Also, as Baler (1965) suggests, in traditional training programs, the students themselves have little to draw upon from their own experience when it comes to topics such as primary prevention, mental health consultation, continuity of care, and so forth.

The training program in consultation must aim toward providing new knowledge and abilities that can be applied in the area of expertise for which the trainee is being prepared. We feel that for one to be a successful mental health consultant, he must have a firm background in clinical areas. However, he must also be introduced early in training to community mental health concepts, especially consultation, as a significant part of the general training program, and the relevance of consultation must be demonstrated.

MENTAL HEALTH CONSULTATION TRAINING PROGRAM IN THE DEPARTMENT OF PSYCHIATRY OF THE UNIVERSITY OF ROCHESTER SCHOOL OF MEDICINE AND DENTISTRY

The Division of Preventive and Social Psychiatry of the Department of Psychiatry is primarily responsible for the training of mental health professionals in community mental health, including training in mental health consultation. The consultation and education services of the Community Mental Health Center Division of the department constitute one segment of this training program. Although the program is primarily geared to the training of psychiatric residents, others such as psychologists (both at the predoctoral and postdoctoral level), social work students, nursing students and mental health workers participate in different parts of this training program. The Division of Psychology of the Department of Psychiatry now offers specialized postdoctoral training in community psychology. A significant part of this experience is incorporated into our division's training program. The staff of the Division of Preventive and Social Psychiatry is composed of psychiatrists, psychologists, social workers, sociologists, and a biostatistician-epidemiologist. In addition to training responsibilities, the staff is actively involved in evaluative and epidemiologic research, supervision of clinical training, and direct clinical services.

Training Program

First Year

As indicated previously, we believe that all mental health professionals should be introduced to the concepts and practice of mental health consultation early in their basic training. First year residents spend twelve months on the inpatient psychiatric floors providing care for acutely and chronically ill patients referred for hospitalization by a variety of community agency workers, physicians, psychiatrists and families. The emphasis on training is clinical and aimed towards the development of skills in proper diagnosis, inpatient care, milieu therapy and the appropriate choice of a variety of treatment modalities. Residents work with teams that plan disposition and follow-up care for all patients. They attend several seminars given by the faculty of their inpatient services in basic clinical psychiatry, psychotherapy and other modalities of treatment. The faculty of the community and social psychiatry training program offer, in addition to the traditional clinical material, an introduction to community psychiatry and consultation services. There are periodic case presentations by first year residents to a faculty member of the community psychiatry group. These focus on the appropriate utilization of community agencies in the care of patients, beginning with their patient's hospitalization and continuing following discharge. Community agency workers are invited to these conferences, and arrangements are made for their participation in the care of patients after discharge. In such instances, the first year residents assume the responsibility of a consultant to the agency workers in the care of these patients.

Through such exposure in an inpatient setting, the first year resident gains familiarity with the interaction of the patient's psychopathology, his home environment, and the socioeconomic factors involved in the illness. Under close supervision and guidance by the community faculty, he is introduced to the theoretical and practical aspects of proper and effective consultation on a limited basis. In time he learns to be a consultant to community agency workers and is able to consider the utilization of appropriate community agencies in the total care of his patients.

This introduction in the first year, although minimal, is essential in that consultation and use of community agency personnel become part of the general attitude developed by the beginning professional. Our work in the second and third year becomes easier since these concepts do not have to be introduced as new and different following a year of intensive exposure to patient care and the development of negative attitudes towards community psychiatry as a less desirable type of patient care. These same opportunities are also present for psychology fellows who are assigned to the inpatient floors as part of their training experience. Under the supervision of the community faculty, the resident is also encouraged to evaluate some of his hospitalized patients' home settings. The resident makes home visits with a social worker and/or public health nurse and collaborates with them in the evaluation and planning of treatment for the individual patient. He is then able to incorporate this knowledge and experience and is placed in a consultant role to the nurse, social worker, or other agency workers in the continuing care of these patients after discharge.

Second Year

The second year of residency is devoted to ambulatory psychiatry and community psychiatry. During one rotation (six months) the residents are assigned to the adult and child outpatient divisions where they are taught to perform diagnostic evaluations, formulate treatment plans and provide different modalities of treatment under supervision. Their didactic curriculum includes seminars in intensive psychotherapy, group and family therapy, development of the normal child and basic principles of child psychotherapy.

The community psychiatry staff is available to residents and faculty for consultation on specific patients who present a multiplicity of social, economic or marital problems requiring the services of community agencies in addition to or instead of specific psychiatric care. Residents continue to consult with agency staff on patients referred to them following diagnostic evaluations.

The other rotation (six months) is devoted to the Emergency Division and Community Psychiatry.

THE PSYCHIATRIC EMERGENCY DIVISION. The psychiatric emergency service is physically and functionally an integral part of the general emergency services of the University of Rochester Medical Center. A second year psychiatric resident is on duty twenty-four hours a day and works in the "emergency" every sixth day. His work is supervised by a chief resident and the faculty of the service. The functions of the resident include psychiatric first aid, crisis intervention, triage and consultation to medical, surgical, pediatric, obstetric and gynecologic emergency services and community agencies.

During the academic year 1968-69, 3313 patients of all ages were served for a total of 4406 patient visits to the psychiatry emergency division. One third of the patients seen required hospitalization. The remainder were referred to outpatient and community services or it was decided that they needed no further care beyond crisis intervention provided in the emergency setting.

The emergency experience is a basic and indispensible component of the clinical and community psychiatry training programs of our residency. The community training faculty works closely with the residents and is available to them for consultation regarding the use of community agencies for disposition of patients and for providing consultation on an emergency basis to agency personnel, police, clergy and physicians. The residents also serve as consultants to our 24-Hour Mental Health Information and Crisis Phone Service that is manned by trained nonprofessionals. This service receives thirty-five to forty crisis and information calls from the community per day.

It is during these six months in community psychiatry and emergency work that the residents become aware of the magnitude of mental health problems present in a community and realize the importance and need of the appropriate use of all psychiatric and helping agency services, the coordination of work provided by different agencies to a patient and the significance of continuity of care. They realize that their expertise cannot be used solely for direct care but that well-performed consultation by itself can avert a crisis and avoid the need for some emergency visits by individuals who are already under the care of other professionals, nonprofessionals and agency workers. Their experiences with patients and consultations are presented in seminars and are used as focal points for discussion and training.

COMMUNITY PSYCHIATRY. During this rotation residents are taught the basic principles of community psychiatry. They participate in a weekly seminar series for six months and in field experience providing consultation services to different agencies.

Outline of Seminars. The following outline shows the structure of the seminar series.

1. Preventive Psychiatry — Principles
2. Sociology
   a. Social Class. A consideration of the concept of social class and of its relevance for sociology and community psychiatry.
   b. Political Behavior. A discussion of the role of individual citizens in national politics and how their behavior can affect community health programs.
   c. Social Structure of Rehabilitation Agencies. A focus on the concept of social structure and its relevance for studying and understanding the operation of community mental health centers, public health agencies and the like.
   d. Modern Industrial Society. A focus on some of the more outstanding features of modern American society.
3. Political Science
   a. Local Politics. A discussion of the nature of politics on the city and county level and the implication of these politics for community mental health planning.
   b. National Politics. A discussion of politics at the national level and how these affect local politics and local programs in community mental health.
   c. The Economics of Psychiatric Care. A consideration of the factors involved in community mental health programs.
4. Psychiatric Epidemiology. Epidemiology is discussed based on data such as those from our psychiatric case register. Emphasis is placed on clinical epidemiology and the use of data in the planning and evaluation of community mental health services.
5. Consultation. Eight seminars are devoted exclusively to discussion of the theoretical framework of the consultation process in different settings and the roles of the different types of mental health workers, psychiatrists, psychologists,

nurses and social workers as consultants. Emphasis is placed on the initial negotiation process with a community agency, understanding the administrative and political infrastructure of the agency, and the importance of flexibility and specific consideration of every agency as a separate entity while negotiating the consultation program. The residents are required to read literature on consultation and discuss these papers in the seminar. Actual experiences in consultation services rendered by residents and faculty are used to illustrate every theoretical point that is discussed.

Practical Experience. Second year residents are assigned to specific ongoing consultation programs run by the Division of Preventive and Social Psychiatry and the Community Mental Health Center Division of the Department of Psychiatry. We want to emphasize that these programs are initiated, developed and conducted by the staff of these two divisions. The conduct and the survival of these programs is not dependent on manpower available from the trainee pool of residents, psychologists, nurses and social workers. A trainee is assigned to a team of professionals who are providing the consultation and education services to a community agency. Initially, the trainee works with the team to learn about the administrative structure and mode of functioning of the particular agency, meets with the administration and staff of the agency and spends a few weeks as an observer without any active participation. Within three or four weeks, however, he assumes the responsibility of a staff member on that team, and the staff member he replaces assumes the responsibility of supervision and training for the consultant work that the trainee does. This method allows for continuity of consultation programs and the introduction of new trainees every six months without major disruption in the programs or diminution of efficacy of the consultation process itself.

Caplan (1965) and Daniels (1966) have described, both from the standpoint of the trainees and of the agencies involved, some of the problems encountered introducing individuals into ongoing consultation programs for relatively short periods of time. The method we use minimizes the problems in that (1) The consultation program does not depend solely on the individuals in training;

(2) the agencies involved are accustomed to working with a flexible team; and (3) they continue to be in contact with the team leaders who remain as the supervisors of the trainees. Also, there are never more than two trainees assigned to any one consultation team at a time. Through this process the agency does not perceive the trainee as someone who is "tagging along" or who has nothing to offer, and the trainee on his part is an integral and active member of the team.

To illustrate this method of providing consultation to community agencies, we would like to describe briefly several of our ongoing consultation programs. The Monroe County Psychiatric Court Clinic is one such program which provides both consultation and treatment services. This clinic is directed by a full-time psychiatrist from the Division of Preventive and Social Psychiatry and staffed by Monroe County Mental Health Department psychologists and social workers who also have joint appointments with the Department of Psychiatry. The clinic also receives trainees from social work schools in Syracuse and Buffalo and psychiatric residents, psychologists and social work trainees from our Department of Psychiatry. This clinic provides diagnostic, consultative and treatment services to the three major court systems in Monroe County: (1) City Court of Rochester, (2) Monroe County Court, and (3) Family Court of Monroe County. Second year residents spend one and one-half days a week conducting diagnostic studies concerning issues of competency to stand trial and presentence evaluations. They also offer consultation to judges and probation officers regarding the care and treatment of convicted offenders placed on probation.

Other ongoing programs available for the training of consultants include a wide spectrum of services to a variety of community agencies. These agencies are as follows:

1. The Center for Action for a Better Community, which is a neighborhood service center of the Rochester program of the Office of Economic Opportunity. Consultation is offered to the outreach staff which is involved in providing care to a restricted neighborhood in the inner city. An education program was designed and given to these workers and consultation is provided on a continuous basis.

2. The Brighton Youth Agency, which is a recreation and counseling agency for the youth of an affluent Rochester suburb.

3. Two homes and infirmaries for the aged with continuing consultation and education services available to its nursing and administrative staff.

4. The Public Health Nursing Divisions of the Health Department of Monroe County, the Visiting Nursing Service and the Social Services Department of Monroe County.

5. The Urban Center, which is funded by the State of New York under the auspices of the Monroe Community College, where adults without a high school education are prepared for the high school equivalency examination, and those beyond the high school level are prepared for college.

During the six-month rotation in community psychiatry, the second year resident is required to participate in at least one and preferably two consultative programs with an agency. Upon their request, residents are able to continue their consultation assignments for a period of a year or longer. We acknowledge the fact that by getting involved in already existing consultation services, the trainee misses the opportunity of learning and participating in the initiation of a consultation program with a community agency. Mutual study and evaluation followed by a negotiation period and consultation program development are vital stages that trainees should have the opportunity to participate in. However, there are no guarantees that new programs will be available, so trainees are invited to participate in initial stages any time a new request for a consultation program is received, regardless of the prognosis of the specific situation.

Following the completion of the second year of training we feel that our trainees have received enough basic information and experience to function as "generalist" consultants and to be able to perform as mental health consultants within the framework of their general practice whether the trainees are psychiatrists, psychologists, nurses or social workers.

Third Year

The field of study in the third year of residency depends on the interest of the resident. Residents can choose to spend two six-month rotations as the chief residents of inpatient floors, outpatient services, forensic services, emergency service and community psychiatry, student health, psychosomatic medicine, and consultation to all other inpatient services in the hospital. While we do not have a specifically planned consultation training program for third year residents as a group, for those who choose the forensic or ED-Community rotations there is further specialized intensive training in consultation. For example, the chief resident in the forensic service offers consultative services to the Family Court judges and probation officers of Monroe County. The functions of Family Court include the intake process run by several probation officers where all family complaints are brought for consideration prior to any legal action. The third year resident spends a minimum of two days a week within this setting and is available for consultations with intake officers, probation officers, and judges. He also conducts group consultation sessions with probation officers in which one or more officers present problem cases to the resident. The resident meets with supervisors and administrators to discuss the consultative process and learns more about the functioning of Family Court. In addition to Family Court, the resident has group meetings with County Court probation officers in which, on many occasions, a probation officer will present a problem case and the probationer himself is interviewed either by the officer or the consultant.

We believe that chief residents' exposures to community psychiatry and consultation services during their first and second years influence their attitudes in training the first year residents for which they are directly responsible. We have experienced a gradual increase in the request for consultations from inpatient floors by chief residents who have received training in consultation and community psychiatry compared with those who did not have any prior training.

In addition to three years of training in consultation which are incorporated into the general residency program, we also have a fourth and fifth year fellowship program in community psychiatry. The fellows at this level assume major responsibility in the training of residents and in participation in consultation programs without the close supervision given to the residents in the general program. Those who desire to do more in the consultation area are given the opportunity to plan and design consultation programs for community agencies with intensive individual supervision and guidance from the training faculty.

Discussion and Summary

Mental health consultation programs can and should be developed for a wide variety of mental health professionals. While the program we have discussed deals primarily with the psychiatric resident, training programs have also been developed in other professional schools and some consultation training is included as part of the curriculum in a range of mental health fields such as psychology, social work and nursing. Programs should also be developed for those already involved in consultation work such as individuals on community mental health center staffs, certain agency personnel, and members of other helping professions such as the clergy, police and others.

The major goal in this training is to make mental health professionals more effective in dealing with communities and to expand mental health services to a much wider range of people. To some degree the inclusion of this training into existing training programs requires a change in attitudes not only for the trainee but for the trainers and supervisors as well. This is one reason why we feel it vital that training in consultation be introduced early into the training programs which are preparing mental health professionals. This training also represents a departure from traditional teaching procedures and calls upon those involved in the area to create methodologies of teaching which will help develop the best consultants in the shortest period of time. Underlying much of this new methodology is the move from the hospital or university into the community and the active involvement of the community and its agencies in the mainstream of professional training. Along with the development of new and innovative methodology, the trainee must be introduced to areas not necessarily included in traditional training programs such as community organization, epidemiology, consultation techniques and others.

Although this paper focuses on the training of mental health consultants, it is evident that such training cannot be separated from general training in community mental health principles and practice. As such, the focus of consultation training should be to prepare the trainee in theory and technique which could be used in a variety of settings and from different role perspectives whether private practice, academic or community based. To include consultation as an important and integral part of the professional's armamentarium, it must be introduced early in his education and not given just to those who choose to specialize in community mental health.

Some models have already been proposed, and some training programs which in varying degrees have been successful in the teaching of consultants have been implemented and discussed. However, more programs need to be developed and more individuals trained if mental health consultation is to have the impact we think it can. Because of facilities and staff, university departments must take a lead in developing these programs although they cannot do so in a vacuum. Community participation is vital for the implementation of effective consultation programs and the utilization of these programs for training.

As mental health consultation is still in developmental stages and there is no unified theory or conceptual framework, it is important that information be shared and communications be open between all of us involved in the development of consultation programs. This can be done through the usual professional journals and through conferences which bring together a wider spectrum of mental health professionals and other interested individuals who have a stake in the future of mental health consultation and its successful implementation in a community.

REFERENCES

1. Baler, L.: Community mental health: Training program in a school of public health. Community Ment Health J, 1:238-244 (Fall), 1965.
2. Bennett, C., et al. (Eds.): Community Psychology: A Report of the Boston Conference on the Education of Psychologists for Community Mental Health. Boston, Boston University Press, 1966.
3. Caplan, G.: Types of mental health consultation. Am J Orthopsychiatry, 33:470-481 (April), 1963.

4. Caplan, G.: Problems of training in mental health consultation. In Goldston, S. E. (Ed.): Concepts of Community Psychiatry: A Framework for Training. Bethesda, U. S. Department of Health, Education, and Welfare, Public Health Service Publication No. 1319, 1965, pp. 91-108.
5. Daniels, R.: Community psychiatry — a new profession, a developing subspecialty, or effective clinical psychiatry? Community Ment Health J, 2:47-54 (Spring), 1966.
6. Daniels, R., and Margolis, P.: The integration of community psychiatry training in a traditional psychiatric residency. Ment Hyg, 49:17-26 (Jan), 1965.
7. Goldston, S.: Training in community psychiatry: A survey report of the medical school departments of psychiatry. Am J Psychiatry, 120:789-792 (Feb), 1964.
8. Group for the Advancement of Psychiatry: Education for Community Psychiatry. GAP Report No. 64, 1967.
9. Hassler, F.: Psychiatric manpower and community mental health: A survey of psychiatric residents. Am J Orthopsychiatry, 35:695-706 (July), 1965.
10. Kaplan, S.: Teaching of Community Psychiatry in Psychiatric Residency Training Programs, unpublished manuscript, 1969.
11. Kern, H.: The new emphasis on mental health consultation. In Bellak, L., and Barten, H. (Eds.): Progress in Community Mental Health. New York, Grune, 1969.
12. Kern, H., Spiro, H., and Kolner, M.: Preparing psychiatric residents for community psychiatry. Hosp Community Psychiatry, 17:360-363 (Dec), 1966.
13. Kern, H., and Jacobson, N.: The psychiatric resident in the community. Community Ment Health J, 5:445-451 (Dec), 1969.
14. Ozarin, L. D.: Experiences in teaching community psychiatry to residents. Am J Psychiatry, 120:271-273 (Sept), 1963.
15. Romano, J.: Engagement vs. detachment. In The University and Community Mental Health. New Haven, Yale, 1966.
16. Sarason, I., and Ganzer, V.: Social influence techniques in clinical and community psychology. In Spielberger, C. D. (Ed.): Current Topics in Clinical and Community Psychology. New York, Academic, 1969, pp. 1-66.
17. U. S. Department of Health, Education, and Welfare: Consultation and Education. Washington, D. C., GPO, Public Health Service Publication No. 1478, 1967.

INDEX